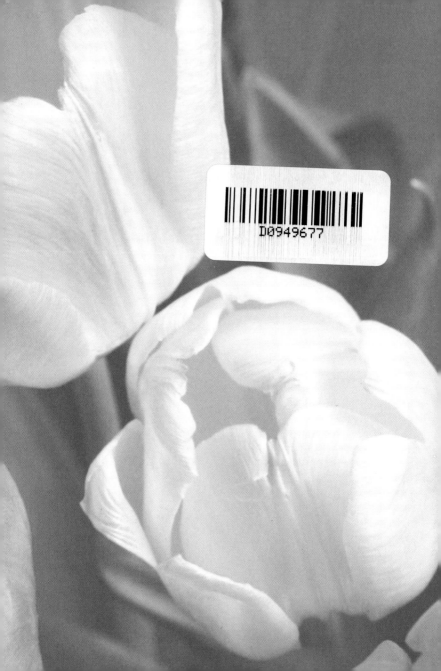

D0949677

The
Secret
Pleasures of
Menopause
Playbook

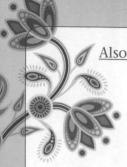

Also by Christiane Northrup, M.D.

Books

Mother-Daughter Wisdom
*The Secret Pleasures of Menopause**
The Wisdom of Menopause
*The Wisdom of Menopause Journal**
Women's Bodies, Women's Wisdom

Audio/Video Programs

Creating Health
The Empowering Women Gift Collection, with Louise L. Hay;
Susan Jeffers, Ph.D.; and Caroline Myss*
Igniting Intuition, with Mona Lisa Schulz, M.D., Ph.D.*
Intuitive Listening, with Mona Lisa Schulz, M.D., Ph.D.*
Menopause and Beyond (CD and DVD available March 2010)*
Mother-Daughter Wisdom
*The Power of Joy**
*The Secret Pleasures of Menopause**
Women's Bodies, Women's Wisdom

Women's Wisdom Web Community

Women's Health Wisdom E-letter
Women's Wisdom Circle

Miscellaneous

Women's Bodies, Women's Wisdom Healing Cards (a 50-card deck)*
*Women's Wisdom Perpetual Flip Calendar**

All of the above are available from **www.drnorthrup.com**.

*The items with an asterisk are also available from Hay House.

Please visit Hay House USA: **www.hayhouse.com**®; Hay House Australia:
www.hayhouse.com.au; Hay House UK: **www.hayhouse.co.uk**; Hay House
South Africa: **www.hayhouse.co.za**; Hay House India: **www.hayhouse.co.in**

The Secret Pleasures of Menopause Playbook

A Guide
to Creating
Vibrant Health
Through Pleasure

CHRISTIANE NORTHRUP, M.D.

HAY HOUSE, INC.
Carlsbad, California • New York City
London • Sydney • Johannesburg
Vancouver • Hong Kong • New Delhi

Copyright © 2009 by Christiane Northrup

Published and distributed in the United States by: Hay House, Inc.: www.hayhouse
.com • *Published and distributed in Australia by:* Hay House Australia Pty. Ltd.: www
.hayhouse.com.au • *Published and distributed in the United Kingdom by:* Hay House
UK, Ltd.: www.hayhouse.co.uk • *Published and distributed in the Republic of South
Africa by:* Hay House SA (Pty), Ltd.: www.hayhouse.co.za • *Distributed in Canada by:*
Raincoast: www.raincoast.com • *Published in India by:* Hay House Publishers India:
www.hayhouse.co.in

Editorial supervision: Jill Kramer • *Design:* Bryn Starr Best

All rights reserved. No part of this book may be reproduced by any mechanical,
photographic, or electronic process, or in the form of a phonographic recording; nor may
it be stored in a retrieval system, transmitted, or otherwise be copied for public or private
use—other than for "fair use" as brief quotations embodied in articles and reviews—
without prior written permission of the publisher.

The author of this book does not dispense medical advice or prescribe the use
of any technique as a form of treatment for physical, emotional, or medical problems
without the advice of a physician, either directly or indirectly. The intent of the author is
only to offer information of a general nature to help you in your quest for emotional and
spiritual well-being. In the event you use any of the information in this book for yourself,
which is your constitutional right, the author and the publisher assume no responsibility
for your actions.

Library of Congress Cataloging-in-Publication Data

Northrup, Christiane.
  The secret pleasures of menopause playbook : a guide to creating vibrant health through
pleasure / Christiane Northrup.
    p. cm.
  ISBN 978-1-4019-2401-0 (hardcover : alk. paper) 1. Menopause--Popular works. 2.
Middle-aged women--Health and hygiene. 3. Middle-aged women--Conduct of life. 4.
Middle-aged women--Sexual behavior. I. Title.
  RG186.N6682 2009
  613'.04244--dc22
                                    2008038100

ISBN: 978-1-4019-2401-0

12 11 10 09   4 3 2 1
1st edition, March 2009

Printed in the United States of America

FSC
Mixed Sources
Product group from well-managed
forests and other controlled sources

Cert no. SW-COC-002283
www.fsc.org
© 1996 Forest Stewardship Council

To the
Goddess
within
every one
of us.

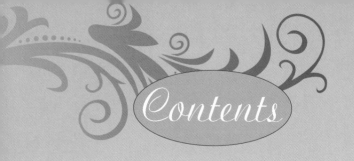

Contents

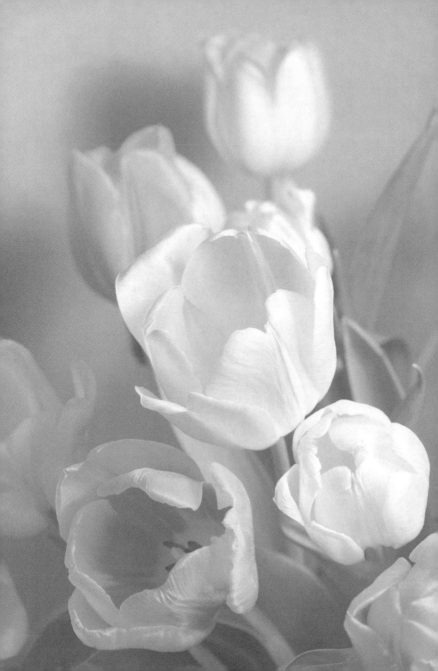

Introduction

Why a Playbook?

When I was writing *The Secret Pleasures of Menopause*, I began to hear more and more stories from other women about exactly what I was researching: how opening up to and expanding joy and pleasure in midlife creates vibrant health physically, emotionally, and spiritually—including amazing sex. I was inspired by the many touching and creative stories I was hearing from women who definitely saw midlife as the start of the absolute best years of their lives.

So I decided to put together a playbook (as opposed to a workbook) that you could use as a companion to *The Secret Pleasures of Menopause*—a book that would provide you with specific examples of what real women just like you are actually doing to enhance their levels of life-giving nitric oxide through pleasure.

These are straight-from-the-heart stories—stories that are warm, clever, poignant, courageous, insightful, energetic, frequently humorous, and amazingly uplifting and joyful. Many are downright *hot!* And all were chosen specifically to inspire you and give you permission to reach for more joy and pleasure than you ever thought possible.

In these pages, you'll meet women with strong, passionate life forces who respect and love themselves enough to speak their truth; heal their pasts; and let go of mind-sets, relationships, and behaviors that no longer serve them. They also don't hesitate to kick up their heels and have a great time, doing whatever makes their hearts sing. The upshot: they've been able to stoke their inner fire and cultivate pleasure, joy, and vibrant health on every level and with every breath.

As I wrote in *Secret Pleasures,* everything we think, say, and do from this point on in our lives will either keep us actively engaged in living passionately and joyfully, or it will hasten degeneration and increase our chances of poor health and disease. The women who share their stories in the pages that follow clearly understand this truth and have undeniably chosen joy and passion. Their stories prove that the pursuit of pleasure is hardly an indulgence; it's a life-affirming necessity!

Let this book be your personal guide to the territory of life-giving pleasure. And make sure that you use the spaces provided (or your journal) to write down and commit to your own personal pleasure plan.

— **Christiane Northrup, M.D.**

How to Achieve Maximal Levels of Life-Giving Nitric Oxide

To experience maximal pleasure (not to mention great sex), you must follow a lifestyle that enhances the production of an amazing molecule called *nitric oxide*. The purpose of this simple molecule, made of one atom of nitrogen and one atom of oxygen, is to signal the cells in your body to stay healthy. It literally resets your power grid.

The more nitric oxide your body makes on a regular basis, the healthier and happier you are. It's perfectly natural, it's easy (and fun) to increase once you know how, and it's the key to developing and maintaining optimum health. Think of it as your secret weapon for wellness!

Here are the six steps to maximizing nitric oxide, each of which is explained further in this section:

1. Associate yourself only with positive people everywhere you can.

2. Eat healthfully, exercise, and manage your weight.

3. Take pride in yourself!

4. Move forward—not backward!

5. Realize that you are what you believe.

6. Understand that sex and health go hand in hand.

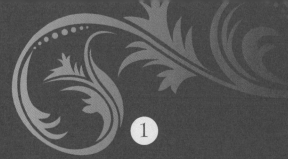

Associate Yourself Only with Positive People Everywhere You Can

*W*e all face pain and disappointment. Stuff happens. But what crushes some people barely bothers others. Your ability to lead a healthy and happy life depends more on your perception of the events that unfold around you than it does upon the actual events themselves. For example, seeing "problems" as challenges or opportunities for growth is an infinitely healthier perspective.

Simply put, your power to live a joyful, abundant, and vibrantly healthy life depends on how willing you are to focus your attention on thoughts, people, places, and experiences that are positive and uplifting.

The following stories demonstrate how many women are able to do just that on a daily basis.

"A friend once told me, 'There are two choices in life: to laugh or to cry. I prefer to laugh.' I concur!"
— **NKM, age 52**

"I think positively and always have. I laugh and associate often with those who do! If you are positive, you attract positive feelings in others. I don't buy into the fact that I cannot do things 'because of my age.' I don't feel as if my life is over; I believe that it's just beginning anew. I intend to love these years (the best ones yet) as much as possible. I intend to live each moment with a *big* smile on my face and spread that smile wherever I go."
— **Irene, age 61**

"I suppose I take the golden retriever approach to life: wag more, bark less. There are just not enough hours in the day to laugh too much, tell someone how much they mean to you, and open up and let people love you."
— **Penny, age 51**

"Being positive is my number one priority. (There's nothing worse than a crabby elder.) I do believe everything happens for a reason, although we may not be smart enough to figure it out right then. Many times what we think is a negative is an opportunity. I concentrate on thankfulness every day, many times a day. The Serenity Prayer is on my computer and the Lord's Prayer is on my mirror in the bathroom. I even told a co-worker that if she had nothing positive to say, then I didn't want to hear it!"

— MJ, age 72

"I want relationships with people of like minds. Time is so important to me that I'm interested only in friendships that are genuine."

— Janice, age 56

"I'm just not a negative person. I try to find something positive (humorous, even) in everything. Even when I was diagnosed with breast cancer at age 35, I made it a positive experience by making as many choices as I could, since I didn't seem to have a choice of whether or not I wanted breast cancer. It really made a difference to my family and friends, and I spent a lot of time consoling *them!*"

— **Claudia, age 57**

"I am devoted to being grateful. Gratitude dissolves problems and brings me closer to the spiritual side that understands that all things are happening the way they need to happen. Every day I appreciate my life, the people around me, and good old Mother Earth!"

— **Kathryn, age 59**

"I meditate first thing in the morning and last thing at night. Before I start my meditation, I say that I love and approve of myself. As I journal and recognize something from the past that wants attention, I write an affirmation to work through and release old beliefs that no longer work for me, such as: *I now release the need to feel* [fill in the blank with guilty, unworthy, unlovable, and so on]. Then I follow up with: *I am a*

loving and lovable, intelligent, sensual woman. I use these affirmations to remind myself that I am a unique being on Earth with my own mission. If I don't give myself permission to do what I believe I'm here to do, who will? This practice has allowed me to like what I see in the mirror each day. Respecting and loving oneself is the greatest gift we can give ourselves and the world around us."

— Elizabeth, age 55

"I use affirmations from Louise Hay's book *Heal Your Body* daily. This has really given me a new perspective and gives me the strength and energy to face my day. My husband has noticed a difference in me and seems to be showing me more respect in little ways."

— Tamara, age 49

"At age 40, I had major issues. I found an excellent female psychiatrist, and what I saw as a journey of a few months to a year actually turned into eight years of painful, wonderful, liberating, rewarding therapy.

I understood things on very deep levels about myself that I never had access to before. I learned to forgive my parents, whom I'd always loved, for their well-intentioned mistakes. I learned to forgive and let go of old grievances, and I finally learned how and when to say *no* or *stop* to others and to give love, time, and credit to myself. This has made me a healthier, happier person who is less quick to judge and less likely to be irked by life's difficulties. One aspect of positive thinking is to plan and *act,* not just 'try.'"

— **Linda, age 56**

"The feel of the sun after days of cloudy weather, the great cup of coffee or tea in my hands as the day just starts to wake up, the sound of the mourning dove before all the other birds begin in the morning, the beautiful blue heron that suddenly takes flight only a few feet away, the colors of new flowers after a rain, the sound of the waves on a deserted stretch of sand at sunset, a hummingbird who comes in close to look at me—I love, love, love these things! And those feelings of love radiate outward. I also believe in gratitude affirmations, such as: *Thank you for this day;*

thank you for my health; thank you for the opportunity to be able to enjoy this moment. Thank you for my friends who care about me, thank you for the relatives who bring a smile to my face, and thank you for bringing me to two beautiful parents who taught me more than I could ever hope to learn."

— **NKM, age 52**

"My husband and I took a Byron Katie course together. The course helped to broaden my perspective and look at situations from a number of angles rather than being stuck in my own focus. It sure has provided a much more positive way of looking at the world and a wonderful way of connecting with my husband."

— **Penny, age 51**

"The key to staying young and having fun is having good, positive women friends to laugh with. I have a wonderful husband, but I love spending time with my girlfriends, too! Women who depend on men for fulfillment and waste their energy making sure that a man is in their lives at any cost *do not* find fulfillment. More often than not, they're quite miserable. So 'girl time' is a big part of my menopausal diet!"

— **Brenda, age 53**

"My girls' lunch group started with me asking a friend to meet me for lunch on Tuesdays. Then she began inviting friends of hers until it grew to seven women. At 57, I'm the youngest. Joan, at 68, is the oldest. One Tuesday, I invited everyone back to my house for a 'wild' party after lunch. I provided carbonated fruit drinks, turned on an oldies music channel, and invited everyone to dance. We all let our hair down and had fun. For at least two of us, that was a real challenge. It was the first dancing I've done in way too long. I like to believe that we have *all* opened up and grown mentally, spiritually, and emotionally because of my little party. We act silly when we get together and laugh our guts out just getting to know each other . . . and ourselves."

— **Martha, age 57**

"I avoid negative news, movies, and so forth. And I'm working on staying away from negative people, including those who are verbally abusive. I try to have personal pleasure, even though I'm taking care of my 84-year-old mom. This has been hard, as I have to be assertive and ask other members of my family to take care of her while I take some time for myself."

— **Beatrice, age 58**

"My deliberate joy has come from choosing to be happy, and making this shift from negative to positive is everything. I learned the technique of appreciation from Dr. Dan Baker at Canyon Ranch [Health Resort] years ago. Find gratitude as soon as you feel yourself slipping because the brain can't be grateful and negative at the same time."

— **Valerie, age 56**

"It suddenly occurred to me one day when I was about 52 that I'm not getting any younger and I had to lighten up. My father, God rest his soul, loved to make folks laugh. Fortunately, I inherited that trait from him. I decided that nothing gave me more pleasure than making people laugh, so I put my troubles and my high blood pressure behind me, and now I wear a smile (most of the time) and never miss an opportunity to tell a joke or make some smart remark to tickle someone's funny bone. Life is too short to be miserable."

— **Paulette, age 59**

"When I'm confronted with a problem now, the first thing I think is, *How interesting!* This makes me stop and take store of just what the problem is and to look at it from a different perspective. Then I don't think about having a 'problem,' but rather about what the solution might be. It provides me with time to make a positive assessment and set my thoughts up for success. This positive attitude helps me gain confidence in myself and my decisions."

— **Pegi, age 58**

"The ability to change a mind-set from negative to positive has actually gotten easier with age. I just think back on all the times when I thought my world was coming to end (for one reason or another) and realize that it didn't. I consciously dwell on the fact that more often than not, what seemed like an end was really a beginning. Keeping that in mind helps me keep negative things in perspective. I know they're going to pass."

— **Colette** (age unknown)

I'm sure you've been inspired to evaluate your day-to-day relationships by reading through these examples of how women are creating happier lives and better health by focusing on positive things—and by spending time with positive people. Now it's your turn. Fill in this section, and commit to more fulfilling and positive experiences and relationships!

My Personal Action Plan for Pleasure:
Making My Environment More Positive

I now commit to being around more positive people by doing the following:

1. _____

_____

2. _____

_____

3. _____

_____

4. _____

_____

5. _____

_____

I now choose to recognize as challenges (and even gifts) the following three things I previously saw as problems:

1. What I thought was a problem: _____

_____

_____

How I can now see the same thing as a

challenge or gift: _____

_____

_____

2. What I thought was a problem: _____

_____

_____

How I can now see the same thing as a

challenge or gift: _____

_____

_____

3. What I thought was a problem: _____

_____

_____

How I can now see the same thing as a

challenge or gift: _____

_____

_____

I now commit to saying the following affirmations
out loud (in front of a mirror) daily:

1. _____

_____

2. _____

_____

3. _____

_____

4. _____

_____

5. _____

_____

I now concentrate on using the following strategies to
help develop and nurture a positive attitude:

☐ *Looking for the gift or lesson in a challenging
situation instead of getting mired in the difficulty
or pain I'm experiencing.*

☐ *Listing five to ten things I truly appreciate and
referring back to my list throughout the day—
especially when I'm under stress or facing other
negativity.* For example, right now, I truly
appreciate:

1. _____

_____

2. _____

_____

3. _____

_____

4. _____

   _____

5. _____

   _____

6. _____

   _____

7. _____

   _____

8. _____

   _____

9. _____

   _____

10. _____

    _____

☐ *Asking for help when I need it instead of thinking that I have to do everything myself.* One way I can ask for help right now is:

_____

_____

_____

_____

☐ *Cultivating a stronger sense of humor and lightening up more often.* I'll list five funny moments or events that always make me laugh when I remember them. I'll think of these often to help me turn a negative mood around. (Having these funny moments to recall when you're having your picture taken will also light up your smile!)

1. _____

   _____

2. _____

   _____

3. _____

_____

4. _____

_____

5. _____

_____

I now commit to taking these actions to create a more positive environment for myself and others.

_____

(Signature)

_____

(Date)

2

Eat Healthfully, Exercise, and Manage Your Weight

To boost your levels of nitric oxide, you must eat nutritious foods (more fresh fruit, vegetables, and whole grains; and less sugar, caffeine, and processed foods). You also need to maintain a healthy weight, get plenty of exercise (both aerobic and strength training), and take the right dietary supplements. In addition, you can bolster your health by drinking lots of water, getting enough sleep, and limiting alcohol intake—not to mention giving up smoking.

As long as you set realistic expectations, avoid being too rigid, and keep your sense of humor, you'll do great. And if you slip, just get right back on track. Don't try to be perfect. Just do your best! Once you begin to see some results, you'll be motivated to keep going.

Read on to see how many women are maximizing their physical health—and reaping the rewards! Then join them!

"Without question, finding exercise at midlife has been a godsend for my emotional as well as physical well-being. When I stay on track with my fitness, I easily feel half my age. My joints stop hurting, I think sharper, I sleep better—it goes on and on. Good nutrition has been more difficult, mostly for emotional reasons. Food has been my drug of choice. But facing those painful emotional issues head-on has helped me make smarter food choices, so my physical health is improving as well."

— **BD, age 48**

"After my mother died in 2001, I took up tennis—a sport I hadn't played since the 1970s. It has enriched my life tremendously because I not only get out and exercise, but I've also made many new friends. Tennis is a great social sport! Now I'm coaching the high-school girls tennis team, and it's incredibly fulfilling."

— **PJ, age 59**

"After selling a stressful business and retiring, I wanted to do something. I realized that what brought me the most joy was practicing yoga, so I enrolled in a teacher training course. Unbeknownst to me, the type of yoga training was power vinyasa. I was stretched literally and figuratively more than I'd been in my entire life. My body responded beautifully—I lost 25 pounds in one year and have never felt healthier. (I also eat a low-glycemic diet of whole foods.) Yoga is truly a gift; and connecting with my breath as well as with my body, mind, and soul has been magical."

— **Marge, age 57**

"About five days a week, as soon as my workday is over, I put on a CD and work out on the treadmill for 30 to 40 minutes. I don't even know I'm walking because the music is wonderful. If I go more than a day without exercise, I feel like I'm dropping into a pit. Regular, varied exercise helps me emotionally and keeps me on track with my eating habits. And to boot, I don't look my age!"

— **MJ, age 72**

"I'm an avid exercise nut. I love classes and intense workouts of all kinds, such as biking, weight lifting, and kick boxing—all to great music. It's the best stress reliever I know of. Keeping up with choreographed classes is also a terrific workout for the mind. It helps me find that natural high. Exercise as part of a healthy lifestyle not only keeps me mentally alert, makes me physically strong, and gives me a general feeling of well-being, but it's also spiritual for me."
— **Pat, age 63**

"In my 60th year, I joined a Pilates class twice a week. We laugh out loud a lot during our attempts to roll like a ball and not like a brick! The discipline of this exercise regimen has allowed me to add half an inch to my height and many friends to my life. It's also helped me bring my blood pressure down. In addition, I walk outdoors with my husband and take vitamin supplements. We eat healthy food most of the time—a big challenge because I love to cook and my son-in-law has two Italian restaurants. I still battle with my weight, but it's better every day!"
— **Irene, age 61**

"Exercise and healthy eating have become more and more important. I refuse to allow my family history of cancer to become my personal history, and I've taken steps to ensure that won't happen. I quit smoking five years ago, I limit my alcohol intake, and I get enough sleep. I also drink very little soda and a lot more water. The saying really is true: if you don't move it, you'll lose it!"

— **DD, age 43**

"When I left my 'real job' four years ago, I put exercise on top of the list of priorities and have held to that commitment ever since. I remember being too busy to exercise in the past, and the toll it takes on my body is huge—pain and stiffness, headaches, irritability, weight gain, and feeling like a slug. Energetic exercise is my medicine. It makes me feel better than any pharmaceutical I've ever used. And it gets me outside regularly, which really grounds me and makes me realize that the universe is in charge—not me! I also feel much better and have fewer annoying symptoms when I eat healthy low-glycemic foods. The big "Aha!" for me was the need for high-quality nutritional supplements.

I never knew I needed them, even though I'd been in the medical field for 40 years! Now they're a mainstay; and the benefits of increased energy, better sleep, and great skin have really paid off."

— **Carol, age 62**

"I notice a dramatic difference after I exercise. I love seeing my muscles become firm and my strength coming back. I also notice a difference in my emotions when I eat meals that I take care to prepare. I don't eat much junk food anymore and certainly no fast food or fried food. I've also been taking cold-pressed flaxseed oil capsules, which make me feel an almost immediate sense of calm. I believe it makes a difference in how my skin looks, too."

— **NKM, age 52**

"Regular exercise—including swimming, boating, and horseback riding—has made me healthier at 56 than I was at 36. I've also worked out religiously at the same fitness center for 16 years. I began with the goals of tone and endurance, and within a month my slender body was firm, and I'd gone from 23 percent to 18 percent body fat! Most important, I felt *great*. My immune system improved, my metabolism increased, and those endorphins made me pleasant nearly all day. Now I do aerobics, too, so I go five times a week. If I miss a few sessions and get a bit grumpy, my husband asks, 'Have you been to the gym lately?' He also joined six years ago. We've both benefited greatly, and I'm sure our increased health and happiness has benefited all those around us. Equally important habits are preparing healthy meals (which means including some proteins with every meal or snack), keeping portions small, and eating *slowly* so the brain has time to register when the stomach has had enough. I never forget my omega-3 capsules, CoQ10, calcium, or my precious vitamin D, to mention just a few."

— **Linda, age 56**

"Belly dance has saved my life, my sanity, and my booty. This practice has strengthened my legs and abdominal muscles and given definition to my shoulders and arms. Eating healthier and exercising gives me more energy and stamina. I'm happier and more satisfied with my life knowing that I'm taking care of myself."

— **Katherine**, age 47

"Nia [a mind-body-spirit fitness program] has changed my life and my mind-set. I try to eat healthy, but there's also a place for chocolate!"

— **Susan**, age 51

"I always go to the gym, and I eat quite healthfully, but I don't consider myself particularly athletic. Even so, four years ago my husband and I completed our first Olympic-distance triathlon! Although I came in last, just finishing the event was an amazing accomplishment. This year, my husband and I along with our two teens are doing it! It's a great family-bonding experience.

Being healthy doesn't only provide my children with a good role model, but it also makes me feel strong, secure, and more youthful—despite the occasional aches and creaks!"
— **Barbara, age 54**

"I read every package for additives. I got rid of almost everything that is processed. I try to stick to really simple, clean food—no soda, one cup of coffee a day, and lots of water. It makes a profound difference in how I feel. My one indulgence is a martini with my husband twice a week! Estroven supplements and Chinese herbs help, as do walking and constant movement when possible (like parking at the far end of the mall parking lot)."
— **Pamela, age 49**

"I started a local Overeaters Anonymous group, and we work strictly with the Big Book. By doing so, we create a community of love that supports us and buffers us from life's daily high and low tides. I follow a diabetic food plan and eat lots of fresh fruit and veggies. I also do Kundalini yoga."

— **Martine, age 49**

"Now that I feel physically better, I'm taking a meditation class to help me calm down from work stress and complete the package."

— **Barb**, age 47

"I particularly like water aerobics. I do feel better with the physical stimulus."

— **Janice, age 56**

"I haven't had a real vacation in years, but when I recently learned about the Sanoviv health retreat, I really wanted to go. My husband didn't, so I went with a close girlfriend. It was quite a splurge for me, but it was truly a life-changing experience that was simply priceless. I loved every minute of my complete health assessment. It was so educational and uplifting, and I learned so much about myself. They gave me techniques to use at home that help me physically, emotionally, and spiritually. My husband told me that it took a lot of courage for me to go, but I was so ready to do something like this that I didn't have to look for any courage whatsoever. I'm so grateful to have gone!"

— **Tamara, age 49**

"I've had weight issues since I was a child, after being molested by one relative and beaten by another. As challenges have come up over the years, so has my weight. I call it my "momma bear size," as it has served a purpose that I finally learned to stop struggling against. Once I realized I was using the padding to help me feel safer, I stopped beating myself up. And lo and behold, I stopped gaining weight! I hit my peak weight, 275, in my mid-30s when I was actively having flashbacks and panic attacks. For the next ten years, I worked on first the emotional side, then the physical, dropping as much as 90 pounds in the process. I hit another very rough patch last year when the mentally ill sister who had abused me died in a fire that she'd started. For me, that meant more flashbacks, panic attacks, and weight gain. But I'm now out of the woods; momma bear has done her job. The weight is melting off, and I'm stepping back into my physicality with more confidence, less self-criticism, and more compassionate self-acceptance than ever before. Thank God for being over 40!"

— **BD, age 48**

As you can see from these stories, there are many ways to add pleasurable exercise, good eating habits, and weight control to your day. These women know the connection between their emotions and their eating. Remember that your attitude and emotions are as connected with weight as are the kinds of food you eat. As you create your personal action plan for healthier eating and exercise, make sure you include things that you really enjoy.

As Louise Hay says, "Those changes that are loved into being are permanent." Don't sabotage yourself. Remember, this isn't another "diet." It's a way of life. So if you just lose one pound per month or exercise once a week, it's a start! Begin where you are. And commit to enjoying the process.

My Personal Action Plan for Pleasure:
Increasing Activity, Eating Right, and Managing My Weight

I now commit to the following ways of eating more healthfully:

1. _____

    _____

2. _____

    _____

3. _____

    _____

4. _____

_____

5. _____

_____

My current weight is:

☐ Less than ideal. I want to gain _____ pounds.

☐ About right.

☐ More than ideal. I want to lose _____ pounds.

I now commit to the following fun ways of staying physically active, strong, and fit: _____

_____

_____

_____

_____

_____

_____

_____

_____

_____

_____

I now commit to adopting the following healthful practices:

☐ I will quit smoking.

☐ I will limit alcohol intake to _____ drinks a week.

☐ I will drink more water each day.

☐ I will get more sleep (at least _____ hours a night).

☐ I will add the following dietary supplements to what I currently take:_____

_____

_____

_____

_____

_____

I now commit to taking these actions to increase my activity level, eat right, and manage my weight.

_____

(Signature)

_____

(Date)

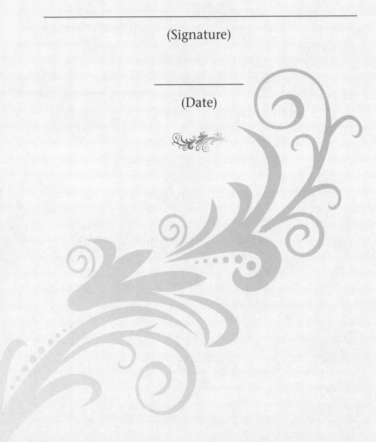

3

Take Pride in Yourself!

*B*ecause midlife is a powerful transition time, it's an ideal opportunity to reinvent yourself. As Dolly Parton once wisely suggested, "Find out who you are, and do it on purpose." Experiment with whatever styles, colors, and fashions feel good and look good, without worrying about what's sensible or acceptable to anyone else but *you*.

Midlife is also the perfect time to reinvent your attitude about yourself—not merely accepting yourself, warts and all, but being *proud* of every inch of who you are. That's the most effective platform from which to reach for maximum joy! And while you're loving the new you, pamper yourself whenever and wherever you can—especially if you're not used to it. After all, you've earned it! Pampering sets the stage for being able to call to yourself even greater pleasures yet to come.

The following testimonials are from women who've had an absolute blast rediscovering themselves—and treating themselves well in the process!

"I've struggled with my weight all my life, but I have always loved myself. I love to look in the mirror, and I even talk to myself. For example, as I gaze into the mirror and smile, I say, 'Girl, you look fine!' Nothing is better for my soul."

— **Janice, age 56**

"I've gained some weight during my perimenopausal years. This—along with my age and social conditioning—has really made it hard to see myself as a beautiful, sexual, intelligent woman. I'm learning to trust that my body is doing what it needs to do at this time in my life. I'm also learning to look at myself with respect as a woman who carried and gave birth to three beautiful children, who has courageously lived through the death of a spouse, and who has had the courage to change careers. Each day I spend a few minutes doing a self-blessing using a gemstone mala [prayer beads] that I made. Each stone represents a part of my body that I bless. The more I do this, the more loving and accepting I've become of my changing body. I'm developing a new level of respect and trust for the changes in my body and mind. (*The Wisdom of Menopause* has also been a major help.) Being comfortable in my new body has also helped me open up to my husband, and our romance has really blossomed!"

— **Lynn, age 53**

"I go to a craniosacral therapist twice a month and attend Pilates classes. I spend one afternoon each weekend giving myself a facial and doing my nails. I get a massage when I can, but it's not often enough!"

— **PJ, age 59**

"I try not to 'could' or 'should' on myself anymore."

— **Pat, age 63**

"People are shocked when I tell them that I started a business after age 45. For more than 20 years, I've been an award-winning medical and health journalist, and I really love my work. But there was a creative side of me (I was an art major in college) that felt unfulfilled.

In fact, I always dreamed of one day being a designer. When I felt myself edging toward 50, I decided that it was now or never. I began designing jewelry and now have a very successful online jewelry store. I'm still a medical writer, but I make time for both and got to realize a longtime dream. The really thrilling part was recognizing that it's never too late to have a dream or to make your dreams come true!"

— **Colette** (age unknown)

"I go on a retreat at least twice a year. The first time I did this, I went for three weeks all by myself. It was the most rejuvenating experience I've ever had. I found a place away from the bustle of the world and went on walks, meditated out in nature, read, prayed, wrote, and exercised. I vowed after that experience to do it once or twice a year. I haven't had the luxury of going for three weeks since then, but I'll go away for anywhere from a few days to a week or so twice a year. It feeds my spirit and my soul, and it rejuvenates me so that I can better meet the challenges of life."

— **Kris, age 59**

"I now refuse to let hurtful comments bother me. I also refuse to put myself down. I've forgiven all past hurts. I love myself more than ever before and can now look into the mirror and say 'I love you' every day!"

— **Irene, age 61**

"I'm a scientist and was a confirmed nerd. And if given the choice to hike in the woods or dress up in heels, I'd be hiking! However, I've given away most of my plaids and have learned a powerful new word—Chico's! At first, this store just scared me. It seemed wild and bodacious, not plain, and definitely not plaid! I decided to try to see myself differently—as Kathy, the stylish one! I'm now a convert and love to wear colorful patterns and fun jewelry—not so much to the lab, but at other times when I'm not culturing bacteria or cloning genes!"

— **Kathryn, age 59**

"I ran a mini-triathlon for my 47th birthday while still 50 pounds over my military weight 25 years earlier!

It still amazes me that I did it. Just to show up in the first place was a huge challenge—so early in the morning, so many elite athletes . . . but I did it. And I accomplished my two other goals, too: I finished upright, and I wasn't last! Out of 824 finishers, I came in 820th. Bravo to me, big time! I look back with so much pride! I've inspired one of my older sisters to take up cycling, and clients often tell me what an inspiration I am to them. What a gift that is, and it helps me keep going and get back on track when the going gets tough."

— **BD, age 48**

"I dress better than I did when I was younger. I make sure my clothes fit, even if I'm in jeans. I want to look my best from the beginning of the day to the end, but without a lot of fussing. I also no longer struggle with my hair. I found a very easy and simple hairstyle that is all my own, and someone (usually a man) compliments me on it almost every day."

— **NKM, age 52**

"It's a lot easier to forgive myself for mistakes now. I no longer beat myself up because I realize that the anger is hurting no one but me."

— DD, age 43

"I use the finest skin-, hair-, and body-care products, which I've determined after decades of research is an indulgence. So are the four fine fragrances I wear, one for each season. Having my stylist cut and color my long dark hair and rid me of my unflattering grays is an indulgence, too. But when Manhattanites say to me, 'My God, darling, you look *gorgeous!*' (which happened today), I realize that for me, these things might just be a necessity after all!"

— Linda, age 56

"I've been more selective about who I'm with. I listen to my body. I rest when I'm tired, I eat when I'm hungry, and I honor myself. I say *no* or *no thank you* more often to my partner, and I actively choose when and where I want to do anything. I used to leave it up to him and then secretly regret not speaking up for what I wanted. Now, not only am I enjoying making choices, I think it takes some of the burden off him, too!"

— **Elizabeth, age 55**

"By my 40th birthday, my hair was pretty much completely gray. Everyone told me I had beautiful hair, but when I looked in the mirror, I simply felt old. I decided to suit myself and go blonde. The new hair color made me feel so much better about myself. I change my short hairstyle often for a different look and variety. My family likes my new look, and people comment that I look like I'm in my 30s."

— **Tamara, age 49**

"Belly dance has made me appreciate my body and see how beautifully I can move. While my husband is supportive and attentive and most of my friends come to watch my performances, some of my friends and family members won't acknowledge my dancing. They think that I'm going through a phase. But I've changed forever! I won't take my health, my beauty, my body, my husband, my life, or my passion for granted again."

— **Katherine**, age 47

"Sometimes when I'm feeling brave, after I step out of the shower, I stand naked in front of my full-length mirror and admire my full yet sensual body as a gift. I try to appreciate all the parts and how they have served me over the years—as well as how my husband still enjoys all those parts! I also say, 'Thank you for this body. Thanks for what it gives me,' and so on. And if a hot song comes on the radio, then I have to dance seductively in front of the mirror. It's great fun!"

— **Barbara**, age 54

"I no longer buy something because it's on sale. Now I have to love it. I don't want my closet bulging with clothes I'll never wear. I love wild, beautiful colors that flow and are fun to wear. I would make a wonderful gypsy! I have to admit . . . there are days when people raise their eyebrows when they see me coming, but I don't care. I love dressing so that I feel wonderful."

— **Diane, age 51**

"I finally straightened my hair after 50 years of frizz. I honestly never thought this would make me as happy as it did! I wake up now to this shiny straight hair that takes no time at all. I look chic and terrific wherever I go. It actually boosted my happiness."

— **Valerie, age 56**

"I've given myself permission to have intimate relationships on *my* terms."

— **Barb, age 47**

"I don't beat myself up for not being the be-all and end-all in my field. I've learned to appreciate *me*

and the things I've done, and *not* compare myself to anyone else."

— **Pamela, age 49**

"For me, pampering isn't about manicures or pedicures or facials—it's about allowing myself to believe that I deserve to be rewarded when I accomplish a goal or achieve something I've been working toward. When I was younger, I viewed every success as something I was supposed to achieve. I chided myself if I fell short of a goal, but I never rewarded myself when I was successful. Now I can actually say, 'I deserve that great new pair of shoes, that terrific handbag, that weekend in the country—because I earned it!'"

— **Colette** (age unknown)

"I buy quality skin- and hair-care products. This has taken more than just overcoming a poverty consciousness. It's been a quest to convince myself that I deserve to be treated well, I deserve quality, and

I'm worth the expense. My skin and hair thank me for it every day!"
— **BD, age 48**

"I went to a Chinese doctor two years ago for herbal help with hot flashes. He is also a master of feng shui, and I was so intrigued by what I learned that I started taking classes from him the next month. Almost two years later, I've started my own feng shui business and have learned how to read Chinese characters. (And to think that I struggled with French in school!) I continue to study because someday I want to be a master myself. *I love it!* I can work for nine hours straight and still not want to stop! It's incredible to find something I'm so passionate about that two years ago I didn't even know existed. I'm overjoyed that I'm turning 50 this year and beginning a new career that I *love!* Midlife is exciting, with endless possibilities ahead!"
— **Pamila, age 49**

"When I left my 'real job,' I got my hair cut very short and spiky. It's now my trademark, and at least once a week, someone stops me to ask who does my hair."

— **Carol, age 62**

"I never used to leave the house without makeup on and my hair done because I thought that I looked bad and others would think so, too. Now I feel okay without makeup and even with going out with not-so-perfect hair. I told myself that if people don't like the natural me, it's their problem. My clothing has also gone from focusing on the latest style to focusing on comfort. I refuse to stuff my body into tight, uncomfortable clothes and shoes just to please whomever has decided what women should be wearing this season."

— **Lynn, age 53**

"I pamper myself with tall, nonfat, no-whip, mocha cappuccinos from Starbucks! I'm their biggest fan. Sometimes I go decaffeinated, but I believe that the antioxidants I get from the chocolate, and the phosphorous and calcium I get from the milk will actually help me live longer—and with great bones! If this isn't correct, don't tell me and spoil the fun!"

— **Kathryn, age 59**

"I take an afternoon nap, retreating to my purple bedroom and sliding beneath my handmade quilt. My husband winks at me and announces to our two dogs that it's nap time, and all who wish to join me climb in for an afternoon snuggle. It's the best!"

— **Penny, age 51**

"I bought myself a whirlpool spa and use it about three times a week. I just love it! I used to feel that this was an indulgence. Now I see it as a necessity, and I don't feel guilty anymore for my 'spa time.' I must keep myself positive and happy for my own sake as well as for the people around me. If I feel joyous, I can give joy!"

— **Tamara, age 49**

"I love my pedicures, fresh-cut flowers, fine soaps in the bath, and the smell of just-washed linens on my bed. I stay in the precious present and indulge myself with the songs of the birds in the morning, the music of the crickets at night, and the heavy fragrance of jasmine that greets me at the front porch when I return from work. The sounds of the honking geese from the river replace honking car horns. I turn off my cell phone, and it's just me and nature reconnecting. An indulgence or a necessity? It's both, because then I see how the universe has truly provided for me."

— **Randy, age 77**

"Being a mom, psychotherapist, and all-around nurturer, it was always about doing for others, but now I'm getting better at making time for me. I work later in the day, so my weekday indulgences include just being alone at home to take care of projects in a less frenetic way and without people around or talking on the phone. It may not sound like much pampering, but having come from a family of nine kids where there was *no* quiet, *no* privacy, and *no* alone time, I now cherish this opportunity. I also enjoy obvious indulgences like hot, fragrant bubble baths and an occasional taste of really good dark chocolate. You can't put a price tag on these things. As I tell my family, 'If Mama ain't happy, ain't *nobody* happy.' I'm very aware that we women are the heart and hearth of our families, and as such, we need to be pampered and respected. I also do volunteer work in my community. Sitting with a 97-year-old woman who tells me about her day or spending time at a youth shelter and hanging out with the kids and listening to their stories makes me feel like my life is balanced, authentic, and whole."

— Barbara, age 54

"Long, luxurious baths with lots of bubbles, soft music, and candlelight are truly a necessity for me as I soak away all the stress. Long, lengthy phone calls with my very best friend are also a necessity. Even though we live miles apart, we stay in close touch. My life would be very different without her in it."

— Diane, age 51

"I think that believing in myself and knowing who I am has helped me make better choices. I make decisions for myself now, rather than first for my kids and so on. I pamper myself with a weekly massage. I also listen to music I enjoy and take classes on spirituality. I get my nails done every other week, too. It's become a necessity for me to pamper myself because I'm such a caretaker to others that oftentimes I neglect my own needs. I need nurturing, and I always wanted my mate to do that. Well, there's no mate, so I do it for myself. By the way, I also buy myself flowers every week!"

— **Beatrice, age 58**

"I go for foot reflexology every week and to a destination spa or spiritual retreat at least once every year. It's a big job keeping positive energy going. Hay House Radio also gives me the daily booster shot I think we all need in this very chaotic world."

— **Valerie, age 56**

"I walk almost every day at dawn on our rail trail, a treasured time of solitude and communion with nature. I take long, hot baths in foaming lavender bath salts by candlelight with a glass of wine or a cup of tea. I read in bed, especially on bad-weather days when I can bundle up and share the experience with our dog, Nigel. I let my husband cook for me and run errands. I have monthly massages. I watch *Dancing with the Stars* without fail. I consider this part of giving to myself, something I can do without continuing to harbor resentment toward those I believe should have given to me."

— **Kathy, age 57**

"Besides my Pilates lessons, which I consider more pampering than exercising because I love it so much, I go for regular massages. After my husband died, I found that I really needed the human contact and touching that this provides. Now I love the flexibility and de-stressing that's part of the package."

— **MEG, age 57**

"Occasionally, I stay in my pj's and sleep on and off all day. Due to everyday stresses, we can't always relax when we need to, so it's necessary to recharge our batteries and indulge in our solitude."
— **Barb, age 47**

"I go out to dinner with my husband. After schoolwork and 'work' work, not to mention housework, I need someone to take care of me! I have a passion for food and cooking, but for right now, we're eating out! The best part is that I don't feel guilty—about anything!"
— **Pamela, age 49**

"I see a holistic practitioner every four to six weeks and an acupuncturist once per month, with additional treatments for pain, stress, and so forth. I spread all this out so that I'm spoiled at least once a week in some form or fashion. Sitting in bed with my coffee in the morning is also special—a slow and warm start to each day, with the sun streaming in the windows."
— **Babs, age 66**

"Letting my hair grow out to its natural silver color, after dyeing it for 30 years, has supported my newfound freedom in just being me. I pamper myself by making time to buy and prepare the best food I can. This is a joy for me, as I love cooking and the creativity that I can express with it. I also try to have some time alone every day, even if only to read a few words of inspiration, take a walk with the dogs, or visit the cats in the barn. All this gives me the downtime to refresh my body and soul. If I fail to take care of me, then I'm not able to offer the best to my family."

— **Pegi**, age 58

"I'm at peace now with how I look. While I still see what I don't like when I look in the mirror, I also see what I *do* like—something I never let myself do when I was younger. And as time goes on, I see more of what I like and less of what I don't like. I think that's definitely part of the joy of midlife. It's not that you don't care. It's that you care more about the things that count and less about the things that don't—and you have the wisdom to know the difference!"

— **Colette** (age unknown)

"I've gone from being very conscious of my appearance as a young woman (because how I looked was very important to my husband); to hiding out in baggy clothes and excess weight after my hysterectomy; to now feeling fine in fitted yoga clothes, shorts, and clinging fabrics. My husband and daughters appreciate the improved confidence."

— **Kathy, age 57**

"When I turned 50, I decided to get a tattoo. My family went wild. I decided to be less conspicuous about it, so I got permanent cosmetics—a tattoo without all the drama. The experience was painful, but the results are great."

— **Janice, age 56**

I'll bet you're just brimming with ideas for actively taking pride in yourself after reading through these inspiring stories. I know I am. What inspired you? Whom would *you* like to imitate? Okay—it's time to commit to doing the same in *your* life!

My Personal Action Plan for Pleasure:
Taking Pride in Myself

The way I see it, my biggest assets are:

1. _____

   _____

2. _____

   _____

3. _____

   _____

4. _____

   _____

5. _____

   _____

I will experiment with the following new colors, looks, or styles: _____

_____

_____

_____

_____

_____

_____

_____

_____

_____

I recognize that I deserve to be pampered! And to successfully accomplish that, here's what I'm going to do on a regular basis:

1. _____

_____

2. _____

_____

3. _____

_____

4. _____

_____

5. _____

_____

I now commit to taking one or more of these actions to assist me in taking pride in myself.

_____

(Signature)

_____

(Date)

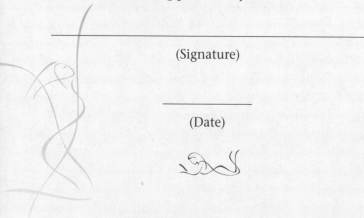

$$4$$

Move Forward—Not Backward!

*R*ebirthing yourself and embracing a new way of life always entails letting go of the past. After all, staying hung up on prior hurts and disappointments prevents you from living fully in the present.

One key is not to dwell as much on what you *can't* change, but to instead focus on what you *can* do. Another is to practice forgiveness regularly (including forgiving yourself), which often involves no longer allowing yourself to feel like a victim.

The following testimonials illustrate these concepts beautifully.

"I had to forgive my ex-husband and the woman he had an affair with for two years before I found out. Our children were devastated, and that hurt me more than anything. I realized that as long as I was angry with him and his girlfriend, it was only hurting me to relive it over and over. I also realized that by letting go and letting God handle it, I could move on—which I did. Nine years later, I am *so* glad he left me for her, and I even hug her now when we meet with our kids over the holidays!"

— **Pamila, age 49**

"I use forgiveness, especially when I don't understand another person's actions. I try every day to forgive myself for *not doing it all* and be pleased with what I can do and have done. I've learned that emotionally, we can't forgive ourselves if we don't forgive others. I've read and reread the book *Love Is Letting Go of Fear* by Jerry Jampolsky many times, and I've passed it on to others. I've had to lighten my relationships to decrease my stress. That's not always easy, but it's needed."

— **MJ, age 72**

"I had to let go of a ministry that I did for my church for more than ten years, visiting homebound and hospice patients. Instead of experiencing the joy I felt initially, I began to feel burdened and burned out. Recognizing this as unhealthy, I knew it was time to quit, but it was difficult to leave people who needed a visit so much. I began to make excuses for not going and even made myself sick worrying about how I would tell them that I could no longer come by. Finally, I called the director of the program and arranged to have another person make the visits."

— **Irene, age 61**

"A few years after a very painful divorce, I had a wonderful love affair with a much younger man. It only lasted about two years, but it helped heal the place inside that feels insecure and vulnerable and not quite good enough. It helped me regain my footing and my self-esteem."

— **Pat, age 63**

"My lessons on forgiveness are daily. I care for my 88-year-old mother and continue to find love and compassion for her. There are days that I'm tested to the max. Before she came to live with me, I prayed unceasingly for guidance. I didn't want to lose myself; after all, she'd be moving into my home! There were many power struggles. I had days of resentment and doubt, and I often questioned my own intentions. But several times a day, I looked at a plaque that I hung on the wall in the bathroom and have learned to live by its insightful pledge: *In search of my mother's garden, I have found my own.* I continue to draw on this strength as her body becomes more weakened. Sometimes I feel as if I'm looking into her fearful five-year-old eyes, and my heart softens and opens wide. Then I can do anything. She gave me life in more ways than I can count.

"I've also had to do forgiveness work around my ex-husband (and high-school sweetheart), whom I've been divorced from for years. For a long time, I held on to the idea that he was my soul mate. As I've grown spiritually, I realized that neither of us could grow in the relationship as it was. I wrote him a letter several years ago and told him that I was grateful for every lesson, both good and bad, that I learned in our relationship because it propelled me to where I am today. I also told

him that I was grateful for his courage to do what I never would have done—*leave*. Years later he developed cancer, and I realized that God had a bigger plan for him. He had chosen a woman to support him in a more positive way than I could have ever done. I knew that if we were still married, I would have been engulfed in self-pity and unable to compassionately care for him during his last days. I'm forever grateful!"
— **Janice, age 56**

"When I cannot be close to people for some reason or another, I always wish them well in my heart and say a prayer for them to have a safe journey in life. This is what I've done for my sister, because we've never been able to truly be sisters. I wish her a happy life, and I wish her protection and guidance. This is how I'm able to love her as my sister and move on."
— **NKM, age 52**

"I forgive my father and myself for believing what he told me as I grew up—that I was 'worthless, lazy, and stupid.'"
— **Michele, age 50**

"I've learned that my time is my own; I no longer have to commit to situations that I previously found exhausting or tedious."
— **Kathleen, age 50**

"I definitely have less tolerance for high-maintenance friends and have deliberately tried to spend less and less time with those individuals. Some of these friendships have been around for many years, so it's been a challenge to extricate myself from them. I speak my mind a lot more and say what I think—something I never did in my 20s. In fact, I've recently been separating myself from a long-term relationship with a friend that just isn't serving me anymore. I feel much more free without always having to listen to this person complain. I'd advise anyone to begin

to disconnect themselves from people who no longer bring anything beneficial to the friendship."
— DD, age 43

"Since age 28, when a car hit me from behind while I was riding my bike, I've been totally paralyzed from the hips down. Yes, I am a wheelchair user. No, I am not 'wheelchair bound'—even though I can no longer stand up or walk, no one has bound and gagged me to my chair! It's just what I use to get around. It's been a constant challenge, but I've learned how to look great in a seated position and how to keep my body trim. (I am the same size at 56 that I was at 19, and it ain't easy!) I've learned how to avoid skin breakdowns and burns, and I manage to deal with a million other details. My ex, who was used to his tennis-playing, mountain-hiking wife of eight years, couldn't accept the 'new' me. He wouldn't go out with me or have sex with me. He refused marriage counseling and eventually demanded that I leave our mutually owned home. *Thank you, God!* I quickly met my newly divorced current husband, and we've been happily married for more than 20 years.

"I slowly rediscovered my sexuality with his unconditional and loving assistance. Doctors had told me that I'd never have an orgasm again. *Wrong!* I'm more orgasmic now than I was in my early and 'able-bodied' 20s. Clitoral stimulation doesn't work, but I achieve vaginal orgasm regularly. Over the past 28 years, I've required some major surgeries, but my husband has always helped me recover quickly by reminding me how much fun we have left to share. I must inspect and respect every part of my scarred yet beautiful body every single day."

— **Linda, age 56**

"At the age of 45, I started on a quest for a college degree. Even though I was working full-time, taking care of my family, and going to school at night, I managed to finish in three and a half years with a GPA of 3.93, graduating summa cum laude. The degree has opened doors and increased my income. And it was fun!"

— **Chris, age 52**

"I have stopped asking for permission. I have stopped apologizing for doing the things that make me happy. I'm finding that the absence of so many things brings me joy."
— **Emme, age 52**

"People seem shocked that I forgave the relative who molested me. I tell them that I forgave him for very selfish reasons: for my own freedom, emotional health, and the ability to attract healthier relationships. I did *not* absolve him of responsibility, but I did do the work that enabled me to stop carrying around the wound, anger, and victim consciousness that permeated every nuance of my life! Only after forgiving him am I able to see the good in men, rather than automatically looking for the worst and fearing abuse. I meet amazingly wonderful men all the time now, instead of users and losers. I *attract* those who are worthy of my trust now, because I let go of distrust first. I had to heal *and* forgive before I could reach this place."
— **BD, age 48**

"Within the past year, I finally forgave my mother for all that I felt she had done wrong to me, both as a child and as an adult. That was a huge step for me. I realized that holding on to my painful, angry feelings toward her would never change her; and it would only continue to hurt me. I acknowledged that *I* was the one keeping myself a constant victim, and I no longer wanted to live and feel that way. As a result, my mother and I are closer than we've ever been. I now see her for the wonderful person she really is and know that the past is the past; she did the best she could with the skills she had at the time. This has also helped me forgive myself for not being a perfect mother. It feels like a great weight has been lifted from me. It's incredible to have all the anger, guilt, resentment, and pain gone— *really gone!* I think it has also made my relationship with my own daughter even closer."

— **Lynn, age 53**

"I'm learning how to deal with my mother in a healthy manner and not argue with or alienate her. I visualize a healthy barrier around me, as if I'm in a glass bubble. Inside my bubble, I'm safe. God has provided serenity, peace, and compassion there for me. As sad as it is to not have the ideal relationship with my mother, I'm glad to have one."

— **Kimberli, age 52**

"Years ago, I got caught up in my family's problems with a drug- and alcohol-addicted brother. My mother loves to bathe in it. I was pulling my own family apart because I thought about it constantly. With support from my husband and therapy, I've been able to separate myself from those two people. My other brother and I are closer than we've ever been. In fact, we're sorry that it took so long. I've basically lost my mother. She and I are very distant, and we act like guests around each other, but at least we see each other and it works. I am overall a happier person. It has taught me that I never want that kind of relationship with my own children, so I'm more open and accepting with them as adults."

— **Robin, age 51**

"I had to let go of trying to control my husband's sobriety. I learned that by trying to control him (which never did work), I was just allowing him to continue his unhealthy patterns. Once I stopped doing that and just started taking care of myself, I got better, my load was lightened, and *he* got better, too! This wasn't an easy process, but joining Al-Anon was the key factor that helped me. I am now a 20-year member and would never think of quitting."

— **Carol, age 62**

"I've had long relationships, and I've had long periods of time without a relationship, just casual, non-involved dates in between. A friend asked me if the reason why I was still single was because my standards were too high. I said that I finally realized that my standards were not high enough and that I compromised too much for too little in return. I've learned to expect more, because I respect myself more. I appreciate the person who has arrived—*me.*"

— **NKM, age 52**

"As I approached 50, after years of anxiety and agoraphobia, I began to melt away the invisible chains holding me back. I learned that my two greatest tools were awareness and choice! Once I became more aware of how my inner negative chatterbox controlled me with fearful dialogues, I could instead choose to change those beliefs about what was safe and what wasn't. I thanked the inner side that only wanted to protect me and convinced it I'd be fine when I challenged my fears and tried new things. I called my negative side EARL because it was Easily Angered, Rigid, and Limiting. EARL roared in my head. But by becoming aware of that energy and learning to quell it, I began to hear the quiet whisper of another force that I called PEARL. PEARL was Peaceful, Earnest, Adventurous, Resilient, and Loving. PEARL was the energy I experienced when I looked at a beautiful sunset or into the eyes of my newborn granddaughter.

"I began to enlist 'PEARL Power' to tackle my fears. Maybe I encountered a few more hot flashes, but the journey was well worth the effort. I practiced traveling farther and farther away from home. I knew I'd succeeded when I flew to visit my sister who lived in the Bahamas. It took me 20 years to get there, but, hey, I did it! I now easily travel anywhere I want. Greece was gorgeous, Hawaii calmingly beautiful, but best of all has been the journey inward to reconnect with my inner spirit and with my life! I even wrote a book called *Anxiety Rescue: Simple Strategies to Stop Fear from Ruling Your Life*. I decided to give back everything that I learned in the hope that it would help others."

— **Kathryn, age 59**

"On my 50th birthday, I told my husband and sons that I was no longer going to plan my life for their convenience. They looked at me as if I'd suddenly grown horns, but it was one of the best things I've ever done! I've always told other women that men and children will get away with as much as we *allow* them to get away with! I took my own advice to a new level and realized how smart I am!"

— **Brenda, age 53**

"I let go of a relationship with a married man that I had for 27 years. It obviously served a purpose, and now I respect myself and other women enough to let it go. Now I want to be open to the possibility of an honest and open relationship with myself, as well as with anyone on the horizon. I want honesty, trust, and truth. No more deception. I give myself permission to move on to something better for myself."

— **Elizabeth, age 55**

"When I was in perimenopause, I went through a phase where I had no social filters. I said what was on my mind, and it was very liberating. I've been married to an abusive man for 28 years and finally told him to shape up or we're getting a divorce. He refused to take ownership for his behavior so now we're separated. I feel sad but also relieved. Right after we separated, I went to Kripalu for a retreat by myself, and it was transformational. Now that I'll be divorced, I've made strides in reinventing myself. I'm more outgoing. I listen to my own heart instead of bending to my husband's will. I've changed my hairstyle, my Hebrew name, and my outlook on life."

— **Susan, age 51**

"A longtime girlfriend and I stopped talking for about seven years. I'm not even sure why she stopped speaking to me, but after trying to keep our relationship going, I just backed off. Finally, I e-mailed her and told her that I forgave her for anything she did to hurt me (whether or not she knew it) and hoped that she forgave me. We're on good terms again. We aren't as close as we once were, but the anger and resentment I felt is gone. We never talk about why she stopped talking to me. It doesn't really matter."
— **Claudia, age 57**

"When my youngest daughter left for college, my life seemed to stop. The overwhelming sadness and loss were disheartening. My husband has a very demanding job and isn't home much. My children were my passion. I did what I could to be an important part of their lives. Then all of a sudden they were gone, and all the activities and events that they were involved in were gone, too. I had to come up with new things to be involved in. I had to acknowledge that it was grief I was feeling and be okay with it. That was probably

the hardest part, being okay with my grief—feeling it, talking about it, and going through it."
— **Diane, age 51**

"With hard work, luck, perseverance, and God, I got out of my financial slump. I now own a business and am self-supporting. This is something that shocked most of my family. They thought I'd always be dependent on a man. I've also gone back to school, something that I've wanted to do. I was accepted to a university after high school, but I was frightened by the culture shock and left. Soon afterward, I met my husband. There wasn't a community college in the city I was living in, so I didn't go back to school until now. I'm very happy that I've been getting *A*'s in my classes. I intend to finish and use my degree. It's given me a new goal."
— **Beatrice, age 58**

"I've had to forgive my husband of 30 years, who died two years ago, for all the hurt and humiliation I experienced finding out about his affairs after his passing. This is a most humbling process, because I wanted to choke the spirit who isn't here anymore, yet at the same time, I wanted to let it go into the universe. I've even had to look long and hard at what my own role in all of this was. I believe we've both forgiven each other."

— **Valerie, age 56**

"I've had a negative mind-set about mothers since my relationships with my own mother and my two mothers-in-law (from two marriages) have been based on manipulation and control. Through the healing power of prayer—and persistent prayer at that—I've worked to overcome that mind-set in order to raise three beautiful, confident, loving daughters. It's important for me to believe that old patterns, just like genetic makeup, don't have to determine my path in life."

— **Kathy, age 57**

"I had a couple of friends who were very negative. No matter what their problem, if you offered a solution, they always had a reason why it wouldn't work. I finally realized that these friendships were really adding to my depression, so I just backed off for self-preservation. You know the old saying "Garbage in, garbage out"? It holds true for your mind as well. I started spending time with fun people, and that's when I realized that laughing is a lot more fun!"

— **Paulette, age 59**

"My feelings were really hurt when one of my close friends told me off. She said some really nasty things, and I didn't think I could ever forgive her. But after a *lot* of thought, I realized that she knew I was strong enough to handle what she had to tell me. So I forgave her. I didn't have to say this out loud to her because it was something I needed to learn on my own. And I'm glad I didn't end the friendship because there was a lot I needed to see to help me grow even more."

— **Colette, age 50**

"It's never easy for me, but with prayer, meditation, and quiet time listening for the Lord to guide me, I'm now able to speak up. When I am guided, I know it's right. I'm able to say and do what I must in a loving, kind, and caring manner. My training in chaplaincy has helped me find the tools to do this. For example, I've had to limit some contact with people who were frightfully negative folks. I put up with them for a long time, but the physical, emotional, and even spiritual effects on me were telling. So I actually told these individuals that I couldn't spend time with them because it was bad for me. As a person who's worked in helping professions all my life, I found this extremely difficult! But once it was done, it became easier, and I also began to see more clearly when such situations were arising. So I choose whom I spend time with and when I want to be alone, and life is wonderfully comfortable and joyful! I also find forgiving and being forgiven absolutely essential to my physical, emotional, and spiritual health. There's a short piece I use often: *Please forgive me, and I forgive you. Thank you. I love you.* Even if it's only to forgive and be more loving toward myself, this helps me in centering and focusing on where and who I am."

— **Babs, age 66**

"My mother died of heart problems, as did many of my relatives. So when I was told that I was going to need heart surgery, I was terrified. I knew I'd have to find the inner strength and courage to do this. Miraculously, the things I needed started showing up exactly when I needed them. I learned that the Shadow holds the emotional situations that you can't handle until the time when you can and that each situation holds a treasure. When I set out, I didn't know exactly what I was looking for, but my journey gave me back a lot of self-esteem and self-worthiness. I went down the hallway to that surgical suite and told my nurse, 'Just don't let me see the equipment.' My family said I was like a warrior. I was never afraid."

— **Randy, age 77**

I particularly love that last story—illustrating so beautifully the fact that we're never too old to update our behavior and move forward, not backward. Of course, moving forward always illuminates the things from our past that tend to hold us back. Expect that. Celebrate it. And continue moving forward!

My Personal Action Plan for Pleasure:
Moving Forward—Not Backward

What three events or situations have happened to me that I've previously considered either difficult to forgive or totally unforgivable?

1. _____

_____

_____

_____

_____

What would my life be like if I no longer held on to that anger, shame, rage, and so on: _____

_____

_____

_____

_____

_____

_____

My strategies for beginning the healing process and being willing to forgive this: _____

_____

_____

_____

_____

_____

_____

2. _____

_____

_____

_____

_____

What would my life be like if I no longer held on to that anger, shame, rage, and so on: _____

_____

_____

_____

_____

_____

_____

My strategies for beginning the healing process and
being willing to forgive this: _____

_____

_____

_____

_____

_____

3. _____

_____

_____

_____

_____

What would my life be like if I no longer held on to that anger, shame, rage, and so on: _____

_____

_____

_____

_____

_____

_____

_____

My strategies for beginning the healing process and being willing to forgive this: _____

_____

_____

_____

_____

_____

_____

_____

What I most need to forgive *myself* for, and the strategies for how to make progress doing this:

1. _____

_____

_____

_____

_____

2. _____

_____

_____

_____

_____

3. _____

_____

_____

_____

_____

In order to empower myself to move forward and cultivate more joy, I now commit to eliminating the following things or cutting ties with the following people in my life:

1. _____

   _____

2. _____

   _____

3. _____

   _____

Fears or limitations that I now believe I'm ready to let go of or overcome:

1. _____

   _____

2. _____

   _____

3. _____

   _____

4. _____

   _____

5. _____

   _____

I now commit to the process of moving forward by implementing this action plan to the best of my ability.

_____

(Signature)

_____

(Date)

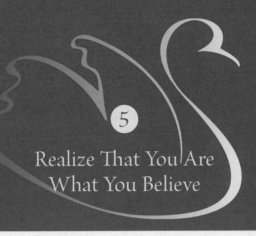

5

Realize That You Are
What You Believe

*O*ur thoughts have an incredibly powerful influence on our reality. That's why it's important to ignore the harmful menopausal myths that keep you from experiencing all the joy and pleasure (including sensual pleasure) possible. So get rid of those old, outmoded ideas and define this stage of life the way *you* want to. After all, it's *your* life. Take responsibility for it!

And while you're at it, feel free to view yourself as the vibrant, sexy goddess you are. Whether or not you currently have a partner, realize that you're fully able to bring yourself pleasure and joy, all on your own. The following anecdotes are from self-assured, fulfilled, and happy women who've accepted that they indeed command their own destiny!

"*Myth:* at midlife you lose interest in sex. *Fact:* my husband and I enjoy sexual relations more with each passing year. *Myth:* at midlife you gain weight no matter what, your skin sags and wrinkles, and you become an undesirable old crone. *Fact:* I am firmer and more attractive now than I was 30 years ago. I've had no surgeries, injections, lasers, or chemical peels—but I do devote more time, effort, and money to myself. Guys half my age are constantly asking me out, much to my husband's amusement. He says that it's a good thing we're so crazy about each other or else I'd be one dangerous cougar!"

— **Linda, age 56**

"I went back to school and got a BS degree and then a master's in a field where I could make a difference. I never thought I could compete with the 'smart' younger generation after years of not 'using my brain' (or using it only to help with the kids' homework). I found that the wisdom of age made me as smart or smarter than the younger generation, and at this time in my life, I could really focus on learning (instead of on boys)."

— **Kris, age 59**

"It's a myth that you have to have a man in your life to be okay. I've been divorced for about nine years—after a 34-year marriage. I'd love to have a partner in my life, and if that happens, great. Part of maturity for me and part of my transformation was letting go of the 'have to haves.'"

— **Pat, age 63**

"I always thought I was ugly because I was born with a cleft lip and partial palate. My mother (and to a certain extent, my father) led me to believe that I was not—and never would be—beautiful. So I've worked on being beautiful inside. One of the tools I've used is affirmations, especially looking in the mirror and saying *I love you*. But first, I pasted this one to my mirror: *I accept you unconditionally, right now, just the way you are*. I'm now operating at a higher level until I just float to heaven."

— **Irene, age 61**

"The 'over the hill' theory is a hoax! I still feel very sexual and more womanly than ever before. I love being in my body, and I have plenty of mojo! My life found greater significance when I realized how precious I am. I tell everyone: 'I am precious!'"

— **Janice, age 56**

"I have two favorite affirmations. One is from a book by Mike Dooley, which says, *Today I am a magnet for infinite abundance, divine intelligence, and unlimited love.* The other is from Louise Hay: *I am always in the right place at the right time.* I like these two affirmations so much that I printed them on business-size cards, laminated a few, and always keep them with me. I really believe that we attract the same energy that we put out. So I put out to the universe what I want to be and what I want in my life. I truly feel that these affirmations have brought all of these qualities into my life."

— **Lynn, age 53**

"I think the whole 'over the hill' attitude of hitting 40 is over. I know that I look and feel a whole lot better than I did ten years ago. I refuse to let friends cry and complain about birthdays. I think if society sees that women in their 40s are just as relevant and beautiful as women in their 20s, the whole youth-obsessed culture might just shift."

— DD, age 43

"It's a midlife myth that your husband might not find you so attractive anymore. I'm keeping myself in physical shape for *me,* and he thinks it's for him! In the process, we have lots of fine sex."

— Robin, age 51

"For many years, the butterfly was my symbol, and I loved and collected them. Then a few years ago, I changed my symbol to a lion, being that I'm a Leo. I had my hair cut shorter and styled like a lion's mane, and I even began to paint lions on T-shirts. I just re-created myself, and I like who I'm becoming now. I'm leaving my timidity behind and 'roaring' like a lion!"

— Martha, age 57

"It gets easier the older I get. I now see my legs and feet (which I used to think looked ugly) as strong and healthy. I'm so grateful that I have a healthy body that gets me around effortlessly and allows me the freedom to do what I want. When I do get down on myself because my skin is getting a little saggy and my hair is white, I immediately shift my thinking to gratitude for how healthy I am compared to many other women my age who are not. I love the fact that I was one of the first baby boomers to reach menopause, and thus have the responsibility to uncover and dispel the myths and to model a new, healthy way of going through midlife. As an educator, I also have a platform to do so."

— Carol, age 62

"My favorite affirmations are *Life is grand* and *All is well*. These are very simple, effective, and meaningful! They're like lucky charms you can pull out whenever you need them. Just focus on what you want—not on what you don't—and watch how it will appear in your life!"

— Kathryn, age 59

"I have positive statements like *Hello, gorgeous!* taped on my bathroom mirror and reminders that I'm in the best years of my life. I believe that each day I'm alive is another day that I'm blessed, and I consciously choose to contribute to a better life and a better world. There's so much 'old thinking' around, and the only way to change it is to rethink a situation or challenge and choose to act as we wish, not as we are expected to. I have a wonderful 91-year-old friend, and she absolutely inspires me to live, laugh, and enjoy life—with no limits."

— **Elizabeth, age 55**

"I have stunning friends who are turning 60 this year; and they are youthful, beautiful women. Some may be grandmothers, but they're not the gray-haired, bespectacled, old grannies of yore. I call them *sexygenarians!*"

— **Barbara, age 54**

"Midlife has become a time of empowerment for me. After a lifetime of being someone's doormat, I'm now an active participant in my marriage, proactive in my health care, and a motivator at work. I share the power with others by being a sort of clearinghouse for bits of knowledge and information that can free others in turn, or I just listen and encourage them as they struggle down their own path."

— **Kathy, age 57**

"I quit a career that I had for 17 years and got my real-estate license at age 51. I love every minute of it! I wanted to do it in my 30s but lacked the self-confidence. It's so rewarding to help people buy a home and see the look on their faces when I hand them the keys."

— **Paulette, age 59**

"I now have a whole new career in ministry as a professional chaplain. I went to seminary and graduated last year at 66, the oldest in my class. I've also started doing handwork again—knitting, needlepoint, and so on—which I'd given up earlier in the interests of doing what I thought I should do. I've returned to swimming regularly, too. I swam a lot in high school and college, but that, too, went by the wayside. My life is still about others but with the clear recognition that I must care for myself if I'm to be able to care for another. My faith is strengthened, my body is healing, and my mind is challenged by all I do today. And the most important part is that I'm aware of all of this in a way I never was as a younger woman. It's just a beautiful time of life, and I shall go on in the belief that this childlike wonder I have in everything that I experience will provide more joy than I know what to do with!"

— **Babs, age 66**

"I meditate each morning and evening, as I've done since 1977. And after each meditation (and whenever else I feel like it), I affirm many things: *1. I am beautiful, I am a Goddess, and I am a perfect and divine being. I see and experience this in all living beings and things. 2. With every breath I take, every hour, every day, in body, mind,*

and in every way, I am whole. I am well—in every quark, in every cell. 3. I am deeply blessed, and I am open and receptive to every blessing I receive. I deserve my blessings and am grateful for each one, large or small. 4. My divine and perfect self resides within me, and God and I are One. God, you are the perfect ocean, and I am your perfect wave. We are one and the same. There are many others, too. Affirmations have enormously improved every detail of my daily life because when said with sincerity and intent, they *work!*"

— **Linda, age 56**

"I became a widow, and all of a sudden I felt old. It wasn't just the shock and grief; it was this idea that being a widow meant that I was old and would be this lonely, uninteresting person. But in the past five years, I've grown so much that I feel younger than I felt at 40. I like who I am and find that I've stopped putting off sampling life's wonders. Friends say that I've inspired them, and although once I would have argued with them, I now smile and say thank you. I thought that I wouldn't survive my husband's death, but I'm thriving, and I love it and am proud of it. For a while, I'd tell myself, *I am strong* and *I am unbeatable.* But now I have an even better affirmation that I got from a meditation teacher: *I am so much more than* [insert whatever is the source of your stress at the time]. It makes me realize that when I look at all of me, there's nothing beyond me."

— MEG, age 57

Nothing is more exhilarating than knowing that *you* have the ability to change your beliefs—and therefore, your reality—anytime. Now it's your turn, like the fearless pleasure pioneers above, to let go of some of your outmoded beliefs and replace them with far better and more health-enhancing ones.

My Personal Action Plan for Pleasure:
Changing My Beliefs for the Better

Myths about menopause and aging that have affected how I view myself and my future that I'm now ready and willing to give up:

1. _____

_____

_____

_____

_____

2. _____

_____

_____

_____

_____

3. _____

_____

_____

_____

_____

The empowering way that I now choose to see myself at midlife (or who I really am once I strip away all my outmoded thoughts and all of society's outdated misconceptions): _____

_____

_____

_____

I now commit to changing my beliefs as outlined here.

_____

(Signature)

_____

(Date)

6

Understand That Sex and Health Go Hand in Hand

*S*ex doesn't just happen below your waist. Sexual ecstasy is a full-body experience and a mind-body event. Because all pleasurable activities, including sex, enhance nitric oxide, researchers now know that having sex (alone or with a partner) creates vibrant health on many levels. In fact, sexual pleasure even feeds your spiritual health in a big way!

The following accounts are presented by women who have demonstrated without a doubt that sexual pleasure is far from being a luxury; instead, it's a vital part of staying happy *and* healthy.

"I had severe migraines until I was 30 years old. They left immediately when I learned how to have an orgasm."

— **Randy, age 77**

"I haven't had a migraine headache in more than six months, my sleep is more restful, my appetite has leveled off, and I'm slowly losing weight. My tension level has reduced greatly, and I've been able to head off any colds and infections within 24 to 48 hours instead of being sick for a week. What I've noticed the most, however, is that I'm happier with my life. I feel more grounded and centered. The release of hormones from an orgasm (even if it's from using a vibrator right now) is definitely beneficial."

— **Kathryn, age 41**

"I began to pleasure myself when I couldn't sleep. It gave me *so* much pleasure—*no* more tension and I could actually *sleep!*"

— **Patricia, age 61**

"Since I've opened up to expressing my pleasure needs with my husband, things have really reached an all-time high for me sexually. I now experience orgasm almost every time (especially with the help of some wonderful lubricating liquids). And I really believe this has helped my immunity, as I haven't had so much as a cold for some time. (Previously, I endured at least two a year.) Being able to truly enjoy all of the sensual experiences from my body improves how I look at things. I have a much more positive attitude and so much more gratitude for all the people, things, and experiences that come into my life. I also believe that this new attitude is attracting more positive people, things, and experiences to me. When I feel happy and fulfilled, I attract more happiness and fulfillment to myself."

— **Lynn**, age 53

"Being close to my husband in many ways—through sex, cuddling, athletic training, volunteering, being with our kids, and so on—all contributes to my sense of spirituality because it gives me a sense of balance, security, and purpose in life."

— **Barbara**, age 54

"I now sleep more soundly and wake more rested. I'd gained a lot of weight while celibate, but now that I have a caring and sensual partner (me), I'm losing weight and not craving chocolate and other carbs as often. I am more in tune with my body. I'd forgotten how to sense its needs and peculiarities. It's as if I've come home to a good friend whom I'd sadly neglected."

— KT, age 56

"The more pleasure I invite, the happier I am; and the happier I am, the healthier I feel. I've found that I catch fewer colds, sleep better, and savor my food more—thereby, eating less and eating healthier. And the more in touch I am with my sensual and sexual self, the more connected I feel to spirit. It's all rather simple. Feeling sexual and sensual keeps me in my body, and when I'm in my body—and not in my head—I feel a stronger connection to the Goddess."

— **Joanne, age 53**

"I think that spirituality encompasses *every* aspect of our lives, so it follows that the enhancement of sexual, sensual pleasure would go hand in hand with enhanced spirituality. I believe that God created sex for both pleasure *and* procreation. I don't have to worry about the procreation part anymore, so bring on the pleasure! *Yeah!*"

— **Gretchen, age 53**

"My quest for spiritual knowledge and ability to achieve orgasm happened in the same time period. Coincidence? Hmm . . . I *do* feel there is a God when I use the vibrator, though!"

— **DCB, age 55**

"I experienced a profound spiritual and sexual/sensual state during the conception of both of my children. My husband and I *always* knew when this occurred because of the intensity of feelings we experienced and the heightened sexual pleasure at these times. I had the same experience during and after the births of both of our children."

— **Irene, age 61**

"Before I began my new journey, I was plagued with adult-onset asthma and cardiac symptoms. I was on daily maintenance meds but found that each time I thought my problem was solved, I'd have to adjust the doses. That was about six years ago. Since then, I've gone through a divorce, been a single mom to two daughters, and entered into a new relationship that has helped me learn (often kicking and screaming) much about myself. I've discovered the true joys of a deep, physical sexual bond. I'm medicine-free and didn't even come down with one cold this year despite the fact that many of the people I work closely with were hospitalized for pneumonia! It's often been a gut-wrenching, emotional journey for me, but my healthy body seems to be reassuring me that I'm on the right path."

— **Carrie, age 44**

"My active, inventive, and playful sex life with my husband has helped me maintain my health and a positive attitude about myself and my body as I journey through menopause. I've noticed some increase in my tension levels, but having sex dissipates that. My immune system has always been good, but it seems to get better with each year. I believe having a loving and passionate partner has contributed to this."

— **Linda, age 56**

"After 30 years in a marriage gone sour, a new and updated version of me has created a beautiful sexual relationship with my spouse with more appreciation for the sexual part of our friendship. My back problems have gone away and my old spiritual energy has returned. I sleep better because I feel like the lioness—pampered and appreciated by my mate."

— **Valerie, age 56**

"I find that sexually pleasuring myself relaxes me and makes me feel more adored. I sleep much better. In fact, if I wake up in the middle of the night and can't seem to return to sleep, sexual pleasuring does the trick. Oftentimes, it will lead me to personal insights as to where and what my tension and stress are about. And it feels great! I also find myself more open to receiving the divine wisdom that flows through me. My whole energy field expands, and I feel more deeply connected to All That Is, to nature, to others, and to myself. My heart opens wider, and I see colors more brilliantly."

— **Deborah, age 54**

"After a messy and painful divorce, I found myself alone and without a sexual partner for nearly four years—a new situation in my life. Lately, I've been coming out of that darkness and am beginning to pay attention to the connection between my health and happiness and my sexual self. I've found a friend who has also become a sexual partner and realized the level of loss that I'd been experiencing by ignoring my sensuality. Now I'm feeling energized and more engaged with life in general, and I find pleasure in all aspects of my life. Orgasms come naturally and more easily than before, which was a huge surprise. My tension level seems to be more under control, and I'm moving through workloads and professional situations with greater ease. It's a godsend.

"Ironically, the physical connection with another person that is so concrete and sensory also serves to carry me out of myself and allows me to experience something higher and greater than the two people involved. Sometimes I've cried after a particularly powerful lovemaking session, yet it isn't because I've been sad or because I've simply released. It seems that sex strips away the layers of protection in which I surround myself and leaves me totally open, totally exposed to another person. I think that it's in this moment that we're most open to and closest to our spiritual natures and to God."

— PJ, age 55

"I have a family history of migraines and suffer from them daily due to multiple factors, including lupus and herniated disks in my neck. My ability to handle the pain of these conditions is very much improved by frequent sex, which I attribute to the endorphins."

— Alicia, age 49

"I have long suffered from chronic pain, and orgasms increase the ability of my muscles to release and relax. I've also found that sexuality is closely aligned with spirituality. Expressing, enjoying, investigating—these are all components of both concepts. Enjoying your sexuality takes you to a place where you're able to tap into a spiritual realm."

— J, age 33

"I used to catch a cold every winter, but since I started focusing on creating more pleasure, I've been free of colds for the past two winters. My blood-pressure readings are lower, and I've lost weight—even those last pesky pounds. I'm much more vaginally lubricated than I used to be, just from thinking about pleasure and fun."

— Anne, age 54

"Since embracing pleasure two years ago as a practice that supports becoming a whole person, every aspect of my life has improved! During my first decade as a mother of five, most of my fun was family based. It took a bit of a shake-up for me to realize that I needed to raise my gaze from the minutiae of my home life and seek a broader definition of pleasure and fun outside my role as a mother. My journey back to self began by reinvesting in myself, physically and emotionally, as a sexual being. I began looking in the mirror again and taking time to shop for things that I loved to wear. I started putting on jewelry more often and getting riskier haircuts that took a bit more time to manage. I also sought out new friendships with women who were already 'awake' to themselves as powerful and sexual. I began to pay attention to what turned me on—not just in bed, but in life as well. I remembered how juicy it was to talk about new ideas with people whose minds excited me. I even started my own small business and made those conversations a part of my daily life!

"I cannot overstate the positive response that all of this has evoked in my husband of 22 years! Like a desperate, starving dog, he was (and still is!) completely undone by this renewed access we've discovered together to my sexual self. A sense of fun and unrushed pleasure once again suffuses our physical connection. Now that I'm getting fed in more authentic ways, my struggle to stay at my ideal weight and fitness level has disappeared. I adore my exercise regimen (Pilates, swimming, and hot yoga), and I no longer look for ways to cut corners. I eat what I like; I just don't crave foods that make me feel bad anymore! I'm exceedingly less tense and have more patience. I believe that my ability to roll with the punches has been upped many notches. With pleasure as my guide and *soft and open* as my mantra, I've found that my health, enjoyment of life, and my family is better than it's ever been!"

— **Sarah, age 44**

These examples are so inspiring, uplifting, and just plain pleasurable that they're well worth reading over and over again. I'll bet that you're now more than ready to make the sex-health connection in your own life!

My Personal Action Plan for Pleasure:
Making the Sex-Health Connection

Physical conditions I hope to improve by dialing up the pleasure in my life:

1. _____

_____

2. _____

_____

3. _____

_____

4. _____

_____

5. _____

_____

After one month of increased pleasure, I've noticed the following changes in these (and other) physical conditions: _____

_____

_____

_____

_____

_____

_____

After two months of increased pleasure, I've noticed the following changes in these (and other) physical conditions: _____

_____

_____

_____

_____

_____

_____

After three months of increased pleasure, I've noticed the following changes in these (and other) physical conditions: _____

_____

_____

_____

_____

_____

_____

I now commit to making the sex-health connection that I've outlined here.

_____

(Signature)

_____

(Date)

Part 2

The 7 Secret Keys That Will Open the Door to Wonderful Sexuality and Sensuality after Menopause

The path to fabulous sex and enhanced pleasure in midlife can be summed up in the seven important keys listed on the next page. You can master these in any order you wish. Why not work on several at the same time?

You may find some keys easier than others, but please realize that they're all vital for your maximum pleasure and vibrant health—not to mention a dynamite sex life. So try to stay open, dive right in, and have *fun* finding what works best for you!

The seven secret keys, illustrated more fully in this section, include:

1. Become an ardent explorer of your own pleasure.

2. Turn yourself on!

3. Remember that a turned-on woman is irresistible!

4. Practice makes pleasure!

5. Recognize and release anger and negativity.

6. Commit to regularly exploring your body's pleasure potential.

7. Live your life in a way that excites, motivates, and "turns on" others to be at their best—and healthiest.

1

Become an Ardent Explorer of Your Own Pleasure

*T*his first key involves paying attention to what delights, inspires, and uplifts you. Whether it's going back to school, getting a weekly massage, taking long walks in the country, or writing a novel, discovering what makes you happy and regularly incorporating that into your life is the first step toward attracting even more joy. You're simply never too old to do that!

Go ahead—buy some sexy underwear, surround yourself with fresh flowers, make Wednesday night movie night, or go away for the weekend with your girlfriends. For even more inspiration, read the following stories from women who have dared to discover and follow their bliss!

"Ten years ago, I found myself sitting atop a retired standardbred horse. Everything in me was transformed. What an amazing experience! I've come to learn what gentle, intelligent, giving, witty, and wonderful creatures these large yet shy animals are! It began as 'therapy' at a riding stable that specialized in such things. But I was so good at it so quickly ('Are you *sure* you've never ridden before?') that I soon graduated to dressage and have a fair share of ribbons. Trail and pleasure riding are still my favorites. And even though I work out, do yoga, and meditate, nothing says, 'Be here *now*—in this moment' like horseback riding. The mind empties, all else falls away, and the horse and I move and breathe as one. And when I'm grooming or just petting my horse, I can tell him all of my problems and he'll listen. Then he'll lower his magnificent head and nuzzle me gently, as if saying, 'Of course, I understand.'"

— **Linda, age 56**

"Several years ago, I decided that I wanted to take sailing lessons. It provides lots of fun and excitement. Now I'm looking for a small day sailer—both the boat *and* the man to sail with! The wind, the smell of the water, the exercise . . . what more could you want (if you can't have sex every day)?"

— MJ, age 72

"The weekend before my 60th birthday, my daughter and my best friend (of 40 years!) took me to New York. I *love* New York. We have lots of family there, but we didn't call any of them. We just had a girls' weekend, doing things that we wanted to do and not catering to anyone! We took in a Broadway show and enjoyed a lavish dinner that we walked off by shopping. We laughed a lot and spread that joy around the city. The experience taught me that I want to do this more often!"

— Irene, age 61

"There's something about gardening that connects me to the earth and Mother Nature. When I plant beautiful flowers and nurture them, my senses are delighted. I've also started growing herbs and tomatoes.

There is an excitement and satisfaction in helping basil, chives, tarragon, and tomatoes mature into something that in return nurtures my body. I also take time for afternoon tea. It's a beautiful ritual that allows me to quiet my mind."

— **Elizabeth, age 55**

"For every wedding, every affair, every event in my life, there I was in that 'little black dress.' While shopping for yet another event, out of the corner of my eye, I spied a little red dress hanging on a rack. Something wonderful came over me, and suddenly I had to try on that dress. I did. I bought it. I wore it. And it had such an impact on how I felt about myself that I actually created a blog called **RedDressDiary.com**. As I now say everywhere I go, every woman deserves to have at least one really fabulous red dress—and the confidence to wear it—no matter her age, shape, or size!"

— **Colette** (age unknown)

"I went to spring break in Fort Lauderdale this year! I'm 52, and I finally made it to spring break! Okay, so it *was* a business-related trip (a convention), *and* I kept my shirt on and didn't take home any beads. *But* I did bask in the warmth of the sun, enjoy a delightful lunch at a restaurant on the beach with an Arabian desert theme, and walk on the beach at night under a full moon. It was absolutely delicious! All of it! I danced up a storm in a conga line and felt the ocean breeze for the first time in 30 years! Since then, I've decided to start saying *no* more often to others and *yes* more often to what I want. I even connected with a few long-lost friends from high school. I've started walking every day after work until the sun goes down, and when I close my eyes, I can feel the ocean breeze and the waves (and yes, even the jellyfish that wrapped itself around my right ankle, which stung for hours) with great delight!"

— **Emme, age 52**

"After 40, I discovered my inner athlete, heretofore unbeknownst to me. I've done all kinds of dancing, road cycling, and even completed a mini-triathlon—all while overweight but feeling great. I took a singing class, discovered a talent for poetry, and regularly use my artistic skills to teach other women how to do their makeup."

— BD, age 48

"I committed to studying belly dancing for five years with a world-renowned teacher and then to performing at a guild amateur event. I told all my friends that I was doing this for medicinal purposes, which I was . . . at first. I felt that I needed to balance my feminine and masculine sides and energies, and belly dancing achieves this with its focus on isolating opposite muscles and moving around a center core of the body. I've gained confidence, grace, and muscle tone as a result—not to mention a wonderful circle of new, beautiful dancing friends."

— Ann C., age 54

"I do endurance riding, which is horseback riding for an extended length of time and miles. I've enjoyed the 25- and 50-mile rides, which take between four to eight hours each. The camaraderie during the training and conditioning rides (about three times per week for two to six hours) is one of the best parts of this sport. I love spending time with other horse people and sharing the peace and quiet with my horse on solo rides. It's a little bit of heaven on earth."

— **Kimberli, age 52**

"A few years ago, I started a book club with a few other women. I've also taken up golf, which I swore I'd never do when I was young. I refuse to take it seriously, and I have a great time playing with my daughter (but not my husband). I also volunteer for four very diverse organizations (poverty advocacy, cancer association, art center, and children's support group). I hope I'm making a difference in all of them and that others see how one person can affect his or her community. I've taken on another volunteer job with a local emergency-services group in town. I haven't worked for money in many years, but I feel it's important to 'work' somewhere in your community every week."

— **Robin, age 51**

"I met a wonderful man after my marriage of 20 years ended. He got me a bike, and we began riding the trails all over Washington, D.C., and had a blast. I was riding 25 miles a day and got so fit! I look younger than I did in my 30s, and I have more energy, too!"

— **Pamila, age 49**

"One of my secret pleasures after a day of gardening is to roll up my pants and put my bare feet and legs into the lily pond. We have nearly a hundred goldfish of all sizes and colors (close to the size of koi), and they suck on my toes and nuzzle my skin for the salt. It's a sensation beyond wonderful to be caressed so delicately and in so many places simultaneously. Who knew that fish could be such delightful companions?"

— **Gwendolyn, age 54**

"My life is extremely hectic, complete with caring for aging parents and meeting the demands of a full-time job. I've found solace in gardening and reinventing my cooking skills on weekends. My creative juices flow when designing where flowers, vegetables, and herbs will be placed. While out in the early morning, I become lost in thoughts, problem solve, envision beautiful places, and gain an inner strength to meet the challenges of each week."

— **Kathleen, age 50**

"While I've always enjoyed wine, only recently have I begun to study the art and science of winemaking. Producing my own is a lot of fun and can be very creative. I share the wine I've made and bottled with friends and family."

— **Chris, age 52**

"I find great pleasure in gardening and digging in the dirt. In addition, I've started eyeing, and even purchasing, yard art. I used to laugh at 'old people' doing this, and now I'm there! Being outside and making the yard, flower gardens, and vegetable patches beautiful and productive has given me a lot of pleasure, serenity, and much-needed 'think time.' To top it off, I left my traditional job (gracefully taking an early retirement before the oppression of an unhealthy workplace would have ultimately driven me out). Then I created a fabulous retreat center attached to my home so that I could do my wellness work on my own terms and on my own turf. If you build it, they will come. And they have!"

— **Carol, age 62**

"Although quilting has been an ongoing endeavor, as of late I've discovered a true creative flow like never before. After years and years of meticulously following the directions to the letter, I'm finding much greater satisfaction in combining all of the techniques in order to reflect the person I'm creating a special piece for. It has also connected me with a number of women, including one most significantly who is 20-plus years older than I am. We e-mail nearly every day and discuss our piecing as well as the pieces within our lives. She's been my mentor, sharing her own experiences, which has often given me hope that some of my challenges will bloom into joys. She's a true inspiration in her ability to continue to learn new quilt patterns to share with me as well as new ways of looking at life."

— **Penny, age 51**

"Travel has been a renewal. What could be better than being together with my husband in a relaxed setting, enjoying each other physically, and feeling young but with a whole lot more wisdom? Traveling with girlfriends has also allowed a lot of heart talk, sharing, nurturing, and *laughter!* Going overseas has enhanced my worldview and allowed me to see the ripple effect of how our actions as a nation and society affect others. It has also increased my awareness of political and spiritual obligations to think outside the box and become more sensitive globally."

— **Brenda, age 53**

"I went to Paris with one of my best friends to celebrate her 40th birthday. She'd always dreamed of going, and we both agreed that if she could sell the car she had for sale and if I could sell some land I had for sale, then we'd go. Three weeks before her birthday, we sold both—within a day of each other! We booked our airline tickets, reserved a room for a week, and off we flew to celebrate the beginning of this fabulous decade for her—a decade I'd already been in for five years in a big way! We had the time of our lives! It was a good thing we did, too, because later that year she became pregnant and had her first child at 41!"

— **Pamila**, age 49

"I started belly dancing during the time in my menopause when I was feeling somewhat homicidal. I needed to exercise to relieve the anger and stress. I chose belly dance because the focus is on the belly, the core of a woman. I needed to be centered and balanced. I've been dancing for two years and performing for one year. I feel free from society's restrictions when I'm onstage expressing the music with my body. Beauty is so tied up with youth in our society, and I break the mold when I perform this amazing dance with my beautiful 47-year-old body. I appreciate my body more now than

I did 20 years ago when I was too worried about what other people's definition of beauty was. My husband is delighted with my new hobby. He videos every performance and is very supportive. We enjoy a more fulfilling love life now that my abdominal muscles are stronger and more flexible. I feel sensuous and desirable again. And it sure has my husband looking at me!"

— **Katherine, age 47**

"I love to invite as many of my girlfriends as possible to a tea party. I put together goody bags, and my table looks like it's in a real tearoom. I serve lots of yummy finger food, and I even wear a vintage-styled tea dress and hat. I encourage the girls to wear hats as well. This year, I'm hoping to hire a harpist as a special treat; it's one way I let my girlfriends know how much they mean to me. I know they enjoy this lovely afternoon, but I don't think they realize how much pure joy it gives *me*—from the planning to the completion!"

— **Claudia, age 57**

"I've always wanted to knit and started learning in my late 40s. I made scarves and hats for my family, and that was fun! Now it's time to make something special for *me*. I also took piano lessons in the last six years, which I haven't done since I was ten. I love to dance, and my next pursuits this year will be returning to tap dance and belly dancing. I have the belly, so I may as well put it to good use!"

— **Barbara, age 54**

"Six months after my divorce in 1998—not yet ready to date but needing a break from my kids—I learned how to ballroom dance. Every Sunday evening, I glided and gyrated and stepped out on the dance floor amid music, human touch, and the joy that comes with moving to beautiful sounds in harmony with another human being!"

— **Constance, age 57**

"Crocheting and knitting prayer and healing shawls has now become a passion for me. I even did some research and found all kinds of prayers to say before, during, and after I've made a shawl. I may not be very religious, but I am spiritual and have reworded the prayers so that I can say them from my heart without any misgivings. The shawls are then given to women who need them—those who've been diagnosed with cancer or other illnesses, who are grieving, or who are staying at our domestic-violence shelter. They're for anyone who needs to know that they're loved and thought about and that they're never alone. The shawls are never sold, but different ministries (usually through churches) do take requests for them. I'm in the process of gathering friends to help with this. We plan on getting together one or two Sundays a month. This way, the shawls will be full of prayers from all of these wonderful women."

— **Diane, age 51**

"Yoga and the spiritual philosophy that goes along with it has been the most incredible part of my 50s! It has prepared me to deal with many of the losses we tend to see at this age. When my husband died suddenly in a tragic accident, I don't believe I could have processed what was in front of me in quite the same way without this incredible foundation."

— **Valerie, age 56**

"I started riding horses in my late 20s. It was a lifelong dream come true. Fifteen years later, I was divorced, relocated, and having to work for a living, so I gave it up. After another 15 years, at the age of 56, I started listening to that persistent nudging that it was time to reconnect with this important part of my spirit. I started riding again last May. I had many fears to overcome, especially a fear of falling, but after almost a year of lessons with a most talented and intuitive teacher, my skills have resurfaced without the anger and need to prove myself to anyone. The spirited little mares that I've had the pleasure to ride have taught me so much about trust, relaxation, and confidence. I no longer have 'phantom limb' dreams about being on a horse's back, and I'm riding for the sheer joy of sharing this bond with one of God's most beautiful creatures."

— **Kathy, age 57**

"My husband died suddenly five years ago, and if you'd told me then what I'd be doing now, I wouldn't have believed you. A year after taking up Pilates, I was asked to do a photo shoot with a professional photographer for the school's Website. I've always hated to have my picture taken, but I have to admit that I've never had so much fun. I've also just started a graduate program to become a school counselor—this was something I've always wanted to do but thought it was too late. I just love it and am so glad that I stopped saying 'If only. . . .' I've now decided that it's never too late to do anything."

— MEG, age 57

"I've stopped putting what I used to love to do on hold. I remember wistfully and with great clarity playing Mozart when I was five, my feet dangling over the piano bench as my hands glided over the silky ivory keys! And although I don't have my baby grand piano (yet), I've started to play again on a portable roll-up keyboard, and I'm slowly and joyfully working my way back to Mozart! It's helped me remember the gutsy five-year-old still within me. We *can* do anything we set our heart on!"

— **Emme, age 52**

"Living just an hour's drive from New York City, I'm able to enjoy being a member of the Metropolitan Museum of Art, the Met Opera, and the Yale Club. My husband and I did this for ourselves when our son graduated from college and we finally had some money to spend on us for a change. The visual and aural rewards have been astounding. And the occasional Broadway show doesn't hurt either!"

— **Linda, age 56**

"I took up golf about six years ago, and it has changed my life. I forget about all of my work and have found golf to be a total release. I enjoy playing with my husband and girlfriends, and I like it when I'm asked on outings with other friends or business associates. It shows who I am in a different light. And I also recently started taking piano lessons. It's more difficult than I ever imagined, but it's fun, too. I've read that it's a wonderful exercise for the brain because it uses both the right and left hemispheres, preventing atrophy. The bottom line is that I finally have some time for myself, and I'm really enjoying it."

— **Colette, age 50**

"I study Ikenobo Ikebana (the art of arranging flowers) after work with an 85-year-old sensei (master instructor) from Japan. For one hour each week, I'm absolutely immersed in listening to the flower and what it has to tell me about how it wants to be arranged. It's an active meditation on how we emerge, grow, and transcend our situation to become the essence of who we are meant to be. It's a most sensuous form of relaxation that completely takes me out of myself—and I get to enjoy a beautiful arrangement for the rest of the week."

— **Gwendolyn, age 54**

"I've gone back to school for a master's degree in theology because I want to be a hospice pastoral-care counselor. I needed a brain stretch *and* a body stretch after putting everyone else—family, parents, and employees—ahead of myself for 25 years. Finally, I'm putting myself first. I've learned that you cannot give if your well is dry."

— **Pamela, age 49**

"I walk to take fresh air and scents into my lungs, as I listen to the crashing waves of the ocean or the sounds of birds in the park. I light candles, listen to music with headphones, take hot baths with oil, get pedicures, buy a new lipstick or blush, get my hair cut, and see matinee movies. These simple treats balance, calm, and relax me—especially the walking. When I walk, I find myself meditating in a way, sorting through my thoughts, and I feel refreshed when I return home."

— **NKM, age 52**

"I'm presently in my third semester of studying Chinese. I've been interested in China since childhood and was very fortunate to study the language for two years in high school. I'm even planning a trip there. I'm fascinated with culture and cultural arts, so I've also decided to retire from teaching but to begin the adventure of Far East travel as a lifelong learner."

— **Evelyn, age 58**

There, wasn't that fun—and inspiring? There's nothing like reading about how others increase pleasure in their lives to inspire us to bring more of it into ours!

Now it's *your* turn!

My Personal Action Plan for Pleasure:
Exploring and Cultivating Joy

Things I already do to cultivate pleasure in my life, and how I could expand on them to attract even more pleasure:

1. _____

I can expand on this by: _____

_____

2. _____

I can expand on this by: _____

_____

3. _____

I can expand on this by: _____

_____

4. _____

I can expand on this by: _____

_____

5. _____

I can expand on this by: _____

_____

New hobbies, sports, or practices that I'm interested in trying:

1. _____

2. _____

3. _____

Classes I'm interested in taking or new skills I'm interested in acquiring:

1. _____

2. _____

3. _____

Trips and excursions I'm interested in taking:

1. _____

2. _____

3. _____

Other ideas or plans for exploring pleasure: _____

_____

_____

_____

_____

_____

_____

_____

I now commit to being an ardent explorer of my own pleasure.

_____

(Signature)

_____

(Date)

2

Turn Yourself On!

he turn-on first requires reprogramming your brain to switch on positive, life-affirming thoughts. To prime yourself for maximum pleasure and to experience the power of your own sexuality and sensuality, start with some affirmations that really light your fire (such as, *I am a gorgeous, sexy force of nature*). Say your favorite one out loud to yourself at least twice a day.

You might also want to read erotic books, watch sensual movies (with or without your partner), or even take baths by candlelight. For still more ideas, read the following from many fabulous midlife women who have successfully discovered creative ways to turn themselves on. Then try their ideas yourself, and have fun discovering your own!

"My daughter hosted a Pure Romance party at my house. Wow, was that a stretch for me! I was brought up with the idea that sexual pleasure was *not* something to talk about or even admit to. At first, I felt very shy and timid. But by the end of the evening, we were all laughing and having so much fun with the 'toys' that many of my inhibitions melted away, and I began to feel comfortable being more open about my sexuality. I even bought some of the products and got the nerve to use them with my husband—something that I *never* would have done a few years ago. Our love life has really improved as we both open up to each other."

— **Lynn, age 53**

"Interestingly, I find sensuality to be less about body parts and more about intelligence. I thought *The Piano* and *Girl with a Pearl Earring* were very sexy films."

— **Pat, age 63**

"We role-play more. When we go out, I often wear sexier clothes. We've started to go to topless or nude beaches for vacation. I love the freedom, and my husband loves the way I look. I also love porn movies! I can't watch more than one at a time, but it does put me in the mood."

— **Robin, age 51**

"I sit in my favorite chaise longue or lie on my bed and listen to some sexy tunes on my iPod. *Sex and the City* was my favorite show when it was on, and now I have the CD set and I love it! Their honesty and straightforward approach was always great to set the tone for getting what you want!"

— **Pamila, age 49**

"A hot bath, relaxation, nice music, clean sheets right off the clothesline, and fresh air from outdoors turn me on—and so does being on vacation with lots of idle time and no particular place to go."

— **Carol, age 62**

"Movies, music, and massages turn me on. And daydreaming."

— **NKM, age 52**

"*A Walk in the Clouds* is one of the best movies for turning me on."

— **Irene, age 61**

"My husband and I are fun-loving, adventuresome ex-English professors, so the list of books and movies we've found sensual and erotic is lengthy and eccentrically diverse! Jane Austen turns us both on! (My husband is Darcy, only better.) Certain movies of various ratings turn me on, then I turn him on, or vice versa. We also play bedroom poker as well as role-play."

— **Linda, age 56**

"Sometimes a scene in a movie, watching dogs mate (corny, I know), or reading a good novel and getting all worked up over the sex scene in the story turns me on. I fantasize for self-pleasure. The R-rated movie *Never Again* with Jill Clayburgh and Jeffrey Tambor was a real keeper, and I *highly* recommend it for any woman over 50. It's *hilarious* and *very* well written."

— **Martha, age 57**

"I like the whole romantic scene—music, candlelight, and fragrance. I watched a pornographic movie with someone else and found it to be a turnoff because of the language. But I thought *Emmanuelle* was erotic. I've never looked at a person's body as a turn-on because the mind was what I was always attracted to first. I have to say now that looking at my companion's body, knowing all the tenderness contained in those hands and arms—even with his two knee replacements—I find in him all the eroticism I need. I keep several of his messages on my voice-mail recorder just to hear him whenever I want to. He is 82, he still has his pilot's license, and I believe he still skis. He is his own man, and that's very sensual and erotic to me. He has stories of world travels that he hasn't touched on yet, and that always holds my interest."

— **Randy, age 77**

"I like reading erotic stories or watching erotic—but not pornographic—movies. There's a book called *Herotica* about women's sexual fantasies. Although I don't like all of the stories, some are quite sensual and sexually stimulating."

— **Lynn, age 53**

"I get my toenails painted red! It's an indulgence, but it makes me smile and feel very sexy."

— **Constance, age 57**

"Fantasizing about being with someone else or others, or fantasizing about watching others helps.

Sometimes just touching and stroking my husband naked gets me going. We find that having sex away from home (whether it's in a hotel, bed and breakfast, or someone's guest room) is erotic. Maybe it's the chance someone might hear us, I don't know . . . or maybe it's because we're really relaxed and away from stressors."

— **Claudia, age 57**

"Vacation venue is an automatic turn-on. I always pack bath oils and other bath items, such as fragrant candles, sexy lingerie, and so on. We most enjoy having sex on the balcony (or roof!) of whichever hotel we're in. Also, we love poetry by Pablo Neruda and soft porn (usually with women making love to each other). There's just something so sensual about a woman's body that gets us both going!"

— **Barbara, age 54**

"I found *The Bridges of Madison County* to be erotic. I was just so moved by the whole concept of being in love with someone and letting him go. I felt her hand on that doorknob and wanted her to open it so badly."

— **Linda, age 57**

"I think about sex and visualize it to get turned on. The anticipation increases as the day goes on."

— **Diane, age 51**

"My husband, a good bottle of wine, and nice music turns me on. What else could a girl want?"

— **Paulette, age 59**

"My favorite erotic movie of late has been *Unfaithful*, starring Diane Lane and Olivier Martinez. I can watch the first part of that movie over and over because the sex scenes are so hot. After Olivier leaves the plot (I won't spoil it for people who haven't seen the film), I turn it off! I'm also a big fan of vibrators and sex toys, to use by myself and with a partner."

— **DD, age 43**

"I can't remember ever *not* feeling sexual. I hold lots of energy and fire in my pelvis. It's what I call my mojo. It always brings me pleasure, and I'm conscious of it most of the time. When I practice bringing the energy up from the earth into my pelvis, it's exhilarating. I love being a woman."

— **Janice, age 56**

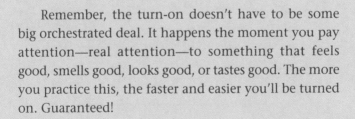

Remember, the turn-on doesn't have to be some big orchestrated deal. It happens the moment you pay attention—real attention—to something that feels good, smells good, looks good, or tastes good. The more you practice this, the faster and easier you'll be turned on. Guaranteed!

My Personal Action Plan for Pleasure:
Turning Myself On

I'll add the following to my list of daily affirmations:

☐ *I make love with unleashed abandon. I am an unbridled, gorgeous, sexy force of nature.*

☐ *I am Aphrodite incarnate. My body, mind, and spirit are wide-open channels for total sexual ecstasy.*

☐ *I am completely turned on and irresistible. I am the embodiment of wild abandon and pleasure. I am the Divine courtesan.*

☐ *Divine love and Divine sexuality now awaken me to sexual pleasure beyond my wildest dreams.*

☐ _____

_____

☐ _____

_____

I will read (or reread) the following steamy books:

1. _____
2. _____
3. _____

I'll rent the following movies or buy them for my video library:

1. _____
2. _____
3. _____

I'll keep the following "mood music" on hand and will listen to it often:

1. _____
2. _____
3. _____

Other ideas (including clothes or outfits to wear, places to go, or things to do) that I want to try because they would make me feel sexier:

1. _____

2. _____

3. _____

4. _____

5. _____

I now commit to turning myself on regularly by following this plan.

_____

(Signature)

_____

(Date)

3

Remember That a Turned-on
Woman Is Irresistible!

*Y*ou'll find that as you continue to practice turning yourself on, your desire will become virtual Viagra for your partner. There is no more potent aphrodisiac on the planet than a woman who feels irresistible. But don't think that only potential partners will be attracted to you. You'll find that when you start stoking your life force in a major way, you'll become a magnet for all sorts of people who will simply want to be around you! You'll have a certain glow, and it will get you noticed every time. Read on and let women who've experienced this themselves describe how it happens.

"I'm told I have stunning eyes, but I get the most attention from both sexes when I'm simply feeling like my lively exuberant self; smiling big, genuine smiles; and enjoying the hell out of my life."

— **BD, age 48**

"Since I decided to put myself first, I've noticed more men being attracted to me. I was caught off guard at work a few weeks ago by a resident surgeon who decided to kiss me on my cheek. He and I have worked together off and on for a year, and we get along well but really don't know each other. His interest in me was a surprise because I had no clue that he was attracted to me. I'm hoping that we get to know each other better."

— **Kathryn, age 41**

"The other day a man in my writing group remarked how good I looked. He commented that I always look great, but that day, I looked even better. I giggled to myself, because I'd consciously upped my pleasure quotient in the last week."

— **Joanne, age 53**

"I think I get the most attention when people see my compassion, thoughtfulness, and positive way. I have a great smile and a great sense of humor. My partner thinks I'm sexy all the time, no matter what I'm doing."

— **MJ, age 72**

"People are attracted to me because of my sense of humor. I am precious and loving."

— **Janice, age 56**

"I believe I get the most attention when I'm being happy and playful. My husband has told me that what he really likes is to see me having fun."

— **Lynn, age 53**

"My partner finds me the sexiest first thing in the morning. He is extra lovable and complimentary. I love it!"
— **DD, age 43**

"I seem to get more attention when I'm excited about something, which is most of the time! I get so passionate about my career, grandchildren, gardening—whatever I'm involved in! It's especially a turn-on for my partner!"
— **Pamila, age 49**

"It's my nature to see the glass half full. 'Carol, you're always so upbeat!' people tell me. They're attracted to me because of my positive attitude and the fact that I'm playful and incorporate fun into everything I do and teach. I'm always on the lookout for fun props to use and opportunities to give goofy gifts and funny cards, or to wear something out of the ordinary to draw attention or make someone laugh. I also have a screaming rubber chicken available 'as needed,' especially for those who have difficulty laughing. My partner thinks I look sexiest when I'm all dressed up! We've been married 40 years, and when he dresses up, I feel the same way."

— **Carol, age 62**

"People often mistake me for a much younger woman. I'm always attracting men in their 30s and 40s! (Ssshhh—don't tell anyone!) I get positive responses when I'm quite relaxed and feeling witty. I have a good sense of humor and can make anyone laugh or at least smile. I'm told that I have a great smile and sexy shoulders, and men like my hair. But mostly it's my smile they comment on, even in passing. In my past relationships, men have said that they find me sexiest when I get absolutely giddy like a child."

— **NKM, age 52**

"Since I started exercising regularly and dressing in clothes that I enjoy, I get compliments on a daily basis—even from my teenage and young-adult patients!

It's hard to feel down when people see me and exclaim, 'You look *fabulous!*' When I smile and say thank you, I'm really thinking, *I feel fabulous!* My 19-year-old son stopped by my office one day and even said, 'Gee, Mom, you look really nice!' My husband needs some work, but one day he did remark, 'You must have gotten a lot of compliments on your outfit today, didn't you?' I think it has inspired other women to make changes that they didn't think they could make."

— **Brenda, age 53**

"My girlfriends all think I'm funny, cute, and zany. And I try to be."

— **Martha, age 57**

"I get positive attention when I'm being myself. I have a natural upbeat energy that people find attractive. I laugh easily and spontaneously. I'm excited about life and what's happening. As long as I'm doing what I love, this excitement follows me."

— **Elizabeth, age 55**

"When I'm confident about myself, feeling healthy, being joyful, and creating positive things, I get the most attention. My face is attractive and I've been told that I have 'eyes that one can never forget.' My companion likes my occasional sass and rather enjoys it when I'm being aggressive, but he most loves my responses to touch and finds it amazing that at our age we have this sizzling thing going on. The older I get, the better life is! A male friend of mine once asked how I seduced men, and I told him that for me, it wasn't a problem—the problem was keeping them away! Many of my co-workers add their ideas to what they think my life must be like, so there's this whole sort of legend around me. I don't want to burst their bubble!"

— **Randy, age 77**

"I think people sense my openness, my nurturing, my humor, and so on. People seem to find it easy to talk to me. Hopefully, I'm a good listener. My husband finds me sexiest right out of the shower, without makeup. He doesn't think I need it—is he the perfect man or what?"

— **Claudia, age 57**

"I have a great sense of humor, which attracts people to me. I can easily make people laugh and break the ice in new or awkward situations. I'm also a good dancer, and I feel sexiest when I'm dancing. My husband loves to dance with me. He also finds my reckless abandon in bed a turn-on. I can be loud, adventurous, and a dirty talker."

— **Barbara, age 54**

"Everyone says that they like how I look and that I seem younger than my years. Younger men have approached me, and I like the compliment."

— **Beatrice, age 58**

"When I'm upbeat and positive, all the good energy comes right to me. The law of attraction is always at work."

— **Valerie, age 56**

"I get the most attention when I'm being honest, open, and attentive. I still can't fathom when my husband finds me the sexiest since he's always appreciative!"

— **Kathy, age 57**

"My husband is turned on by me all the time, which amazes me after 38 years of marriage. He's a saint. It's so wonderful to know that you're loved and adored 100 percent. But I think men in general are attracted to me for my personality. People are just attracted to those who make them feel good."

— **Paulette, age 59**

"I still turn heads, and I think it's because I just exude sexiness. I feel sexy, so I think others can feel it, too. I'm not thin, but I do have some nice curves. It's fun!"

— **Colette, age 50**

Can you imagine yourself being more irresistible now? Aren't you feeling excited about the possibilities? Remember, you were born to be irresistible in a particular way that only you can experience. The world is waiting!

My Personal Action Plan for Pleasure:
Feeling Irresistible

The next five times I receive a compliment or otherwise get positive attention from others (whether from strangers or friends and family), I'll record here what I was doing, wearing, saying, or thinking (and how I was doing, wearing, saying, or thinking it) that most likely inspired the positive attention:

1. _____

_____

2. _____

_____

3. _____

_____

4. _____

_____

5. _____

_____

I now commit to feeling irresistible—in the ways I just described.

_____

(Signature)

_____

(Date)

4

Practice Makes Pleasure!

I hate the word *masturbation*. It has such heavy, shameful connotations. I prefer the term used in ancient Taoist literature: *self-cultivation*. Self-cultivation and self-pleasuring imply nothing but positive growth, delight, amusement, and satisfaction.

But what it all comes down to is practice. It's the only way you can discover what really turns you on. And it's an empowering *health* practice—just like meditating or exercising. So practice on a regular basis—twice a week, at least! Explore what you like and what works best for you. Experiment with different touches, different fantasies, and even different erogenous zones.

The following accounts are from women who have discovered that practice indeed makes perfect . . . *perfect pleasure!*

"I've been learning how to 'drive my own car' big time. I feel like a goddess!"

— **NMF, age 57**

"I've been doing a bit of self-pleasuring with an exploratory approach: not always to reach orgasm, but to figure out what I really like and just enjoy that. I've discovered that this has actually improved my enjoyment and frequency of sex with my husband. And self-pleasuring definitely improves my sleep!"

— **Anne, age 54**

"I'm comfortable about self-pleasuring. I definitely see it as a health issue and can really feel the benefits to my entire body."

— **Carol, age 62**

"I had to wade through a lot of sexual-abuse issues before I realized that I was chronically clenching my pelvic muscles. I enjoyed sex but wasn't orgasmic until my early 40s. Since then, I'm amazed by the strength and depth of the orgasms I've been able to have on my own with a dildo and a vibrator."

— BD, age 48

"Every woman should have a drawer full of sex toys, vibrators, and so on. I don't know any women over 40 who don't own at least one sexual device. Learning how to pleasure yourself is vital to being able to explain what you like to someone else. Anyone who feels that this is bad or dirty needs to shift their thinking."

— DD, age 43

"I'm comfortable pleasuring myself. My husband travels a lot, and I'm not interested in another man."

— Robin, age 51

"My girlfriends crack up whenever I tell them where to go, what vibrator works, and how! I don't have to wait for my partner if I'm in need of an orgasm just because I want one at 3:00 in the afternoon while I'm home alone!"
— **Pamila, age 49**

"You need to use it, or you definitely lose it."
— **NKM, age 52**

"Self-pleasuring is vital because it's made me more aware of what turns me on, thus helping my husband. I believe that pleasuring myself has helped make me more open to the pleasure that he gives me."
— **Linda, age 56**

"You can't love others without first loving yourself, and that includes being comfortable with your body. Although I thoroughly enjoy sex with my husband, sometimes it's relaxing to experience sexual stimulation and orgasm without having to pleasure him or sleep in a wet spot!"

— **Brenda, age 53**

"It's taken me most of my life to free myself from the guilt associated with pleasuring myself sexually, but I find that it helps me by releasing pent-up tension. I was in my mid-50s when I bought my first sex toy."

— **Martha, age 57**

"I think every woman needs to find out for herself what gives her sexual pleasure. Men often don't know what to do, and so they think that because they're fulfilled (by intercourse especially), their partners are, too. Think again! Also, sometimes self-pleasuring is just a release for stress and has nothing to do with the performance of your significant other."

— **Claudia, age 57**

"I definitely feel good about pleasuring myself. In fact, because of some difficulties my husband has had, that is the only way I've been able to orgasm. I love orgasms. My oldest daughter has given me a wonderful vibrator, which I love."

— **Diane, age 51**

"I found an incredible vibrator at Good Vibrations, and I'm comfortable using it. It keeps me knowing that I'm still in the ball game. I've also turned lots of friends on to it! We giggle like little kids as we send instant messages on the computer at night about the names we've given this thing."

— **Valerie, age 56**

"Self-pleasuring is a natural part of who we are. When we're thirsty, we take a drink. When we're hungry, we eat. When we're turned on, why not follow that wonderful feeling through to the natural end? It's had a positive effect on my relationship because we both feel wonderful, and sometimes it gets another session started because pleasuring myself is very exciting for my partner to watch. Sex is a selfish *and* a sharing act. Both people should get the maximum amount of enjoyment from it."

— **Elizabeth, age 55**

I hope this section turned around any negative programming you might have received from your family members or culture about self-pleasuring. I also hope that it has freed you to begin really getting to know your pleasure profile up-close and personally!

My Personal Action Plan for Pleasure:
Practicing Self-Cultivation

I now commit to exploring my own pleasure through practicing self-cultivation at least two times a week. If I need to release any guilt about this practice (because of my family's or society's attitudes about this), I commit to taking the following actions to successfully do that: _____

_____

_____

_____

My plan for practicing self-cultivation and exploring my own sensual, sexual pleasure (including fantasies to test-drive, erogenous zones to explore, toys to try, and so on) includes:_____

_____

_____

_____

I commit to practicing self-cultivation and feeling more pleasure as outlined here.

_____
(Signature)

_____
(Date)

5

Recognize and Release
Anger and Negativity

*C*ultivating pleasure and joy doesn't mean ignoring negative emotions. They're a part of life. The trick is not to get stuck in negativity when they surface. Feel the emotions; use them constructively to change whatever is needed; and then *let go* of the anger, doubt, or resentment. Having an exit plan ready is helpful: call a friend, go for a walk, play with your dog, or put on some fun music and dance around the room.

Major losses (such as a divorce or death) may require that you stay with your feelings for a while before you can truly release them—as the saying goes, you must feel it to heal it. But even then, find some ways of bringing joy and pleasure into your life as you work things out. Be good to yourself, *especially* when you're dealing with something difficult.

The bottom line with negativity is that you're either part of the problem or part of the solution. And as the following women illustrate, the most effective way to be part of the solution is to rise above the level of the problem.

"I listen to music and sing—or at least try to sing. I don't sing well, but I can sing with all the gusto of Aretha Franklin. (My apologies to Ms. Franklin.)"
— **Evelyn, age 58**

"I've learned the difference between saying sorry and actually being sorry, as well as the difference between 'I forgive' and feeling the lightness that comes when the anger is *really* gone. That is truly a process and cannot be forced. In the meantime, I try to be open and honest about my feelings, and then I take them to a kickboxing class!"
— **Pat, age 63**

"There are times I start to 'awfulize,' which is what I call seeing things in a negative light or carrying a thought to the extreme worst-case scenario. Now I'll catch myself, smile, and get back on track with reality and my positive perspective on things. Sometimes I write in my journal until I'm empty, then I tear the page out and burn it. The negativity goes away."

— **Kimberli, age 52**

"I release anger through verbal jokes. For example, if a man agitates me, I say, 'If I could take him home with me for about four days, I could cure him!' Then I start to laugh. When people question me about that, I elaborate on just what I'd do to cure him!"

— **Janice, age 56**

"I work out or go for a long, fast walk. I need to be alone. Sometimes I scream really loud just once, and then I feel better. A good cry works, too."

— **Robin, age 51**

"When I fall into a distressing mind loop of worry or negativity, I always tell myself: *I have the power to change this thought.* It usually works to get my mind off the problem. The ability to stop the negative mind loop is huge. I refuse to let worry or anxiety rule my life."

— DD, age 43

"I clean house! Somehow I feel that when my surroundings are clean and in shape, the rest of my life will be as well. It also allows me to vent! I can really take my anger out with the vacuum! I can tell people off, cry, hit the couch cushions, and not hurt anyone (except maybe the vacuum). And I get a good physical workout. I really work up a sweat cleaning, and many times I come up with some good solutions."

— Lynn, age 53

"The breathing practice called *pranayama* is the single-most effective action I've ever found for taking the wind out of any negativity. But anything else that makes me breathe deeply (such as dancing, hard bike rides, batting cages, singing, combing the kitty, sticking my nose in roses, or just helping someone else who's in a worse place than me) works, too. A good primal yell—one only, and not directed at anyone—works as well, as does lots and lots of writing. There's no way to overstate the value of learning to change a negative state to a positive one!"

— BD, age 48

"I believe in seeing the cup always half full. Whenever my family or friends are upset about something or clients are feeling angst and want to pour all their sadness on me, I listen and respond. Then I go to a spot where I'm alone and ask the universe to help me release all that isn't of light. I refill by listening to my favorite music, fixing my favorite food or drink, and sitting in my favorite chair to read something of joy! I also had to learn that just because I was growing, it didn't mean that I could impose my knowledge on everyone around me. If they asked and wanted to know, I could share. Otherwise, I realized that it wasn't their time yet, and it will come to them when they ask!

When I'm angry, I breathe deeply and remind myself that my anger only hurts me—not the person I'm upset with."
— **Pamila, age 49**

"I rarely feel anger, but on the occasions when I do, I'll walk through my neighborhood until I can think clearly and rationally."
— **Kathleen, age 50**

"I dance, run, walk, hike, scream, or laugh. I see my ability to choose in the moment whether I want to feel good or bad about a given situation. I keep an empowering context to all situations that I find myself in."
— **Michele, age 50**

"I know what negative feels like, and I don't like it. When I start hearing myself use negative language,

I'm aware of it and tell myself: *Stop it right now.* My husband also reminds me when I'm negative, and that's helpful. Sometimes I get out of the house and work in the garden, or I go to the gym and exercise it out of my system. Sometimes I talk it out. It's my nature to be positive, but I believe you can also practice making the shift over from negative to positive and learn how to do it effectively."

— **Carol, age 62**

"I try to be alone when I have a negative mind-set, and I work hard to pull myself out of it quickly. Sometimes I call a close friend and ask if I can vent a bit. I usually get a laugh out of my friend and a positive response such as, 'Sure! Lay it on me!' But I don't stay in that mind-set for very long. I take flaxseed-oil capsules if I really feel negative or frustrated. Exercise works, too, and music always pulls me out of any funk. I burn incense, put on the headphones, and turn it up loud! Sometimes I listen to Led Zeppelin or anything rock; other times it's Yanni, Andreas Vollenweider, or Andrea Bocelli. I imagine myself as a great dancer, a great vocalist, a great businessperson—very successful in whatever line of work I daydream myself into. After a few minutes, I'm feeling uplifted. Music washes it all away and opens the creative juices in my mind, and I forget what it was that made me feel so negative."

— **NKM, age 52**

"When I take my dogs out for a 'sniff 'n' pee' walk in the evenings, I often vent my anger and dissatisfaction with my husband and our situation or just my frustrations in general. I let it all out to the universe and talk to God. I cry often, if I need the release. I scream, throw a fit, and even create a language all my own to keep from cursing so that I won't bring any more negativity into the situation than there already is."

— **Martha, age 57**

"I realize that being in a state of anger isn't a healthy place to stay for long. Laughter at the absurdity of the situation helps me put it in perspective. Usually anger is a way of controlling, so I look for a better way of dealing with it. I ask myself, *Why am I upset? Is it that*

important? Am I holding on to a need to be right? Why? Then I try to let it go instead. Likewise, when I find myself having a pity party, I try to reach for a better feeling. I check to see if I can do something about it, and I start counting my blessings. I also focus outward, seeing where I can help another. It's amazing how self-absorbed we can get. What good does it do? The value in being able to make the shift improves everything. It expands me."

— Elizabeth, age 55

"Beating my pillows and throwing a fit when I'm alone has really helped me. Also learning how to do the energy-tapping technique that they teach at Sanoviv Medical Institute in Baja California has definitely helped me release anger and negative emotions so that I can be more balanced."

— Tamara, age 49

"I don't get angry often, but when I do, I can listen to music or turn on my fountain and let the sound of the falling water heal me. I also have wind chimes that are soothing and help me release anger. Watching funny movies or saying affirmations works, too."

— **Randy, age 77**

"My mantra is the Hebrew Shema. It gives me strength. I tell myself not to sweat the small stuff and not to engage when my husband gets angry. These things plus meditation, hot baths, and exercise have helped keep me calm and happy."

— **Susan, age 51**

"I'm big on venting, so I usually talk it to death. My husband most often gets to listen to me rant and rave (since it's *not* about him). I just get it all out and can then let pleasure back in."

— **Claudia, 57**

"I come from hot-tempered stock, so I'm quick to anger when I'm hungry, tired, or stressed—just like an infant! I find sometimes that cursing and using violent language (which is ludicrous because I'm *such* a nonviolent person) takes that dangerous edge off. It's laughable to the people around me (who know me), because it's so far from who I am. The release may sound unorthodox, but it feels really good! As a therapist, I'm a bit biased in that I always rely on the power of talking. That may be to my own therapist, my husband, a trusted friend, or someone I think may be there to hear me and really understand. When I'm feeling depressed or bad about myself in some way, getting another perspective usually helps. Also I find that exercise, especially dancing, usually does the trick to get those feel-good endorphins going!"

— **Barbara, age 54**

"I use pranayama and breathe, breathe, breathe. I've learned to send negative people to the light. I give it up and out to the forces that be. I seek to not become attached to the negative energy, as I will only suffer with it."

— **Valerie, age 56**

"I don't allow the negativity of family members to drag me down. I leave their presence!"

— **Kathy, age 57**

"I'm still working on releasing anger when I feel it. But now that I like myself and feel more content within *and* with myself, I realize that I don't get angry so easily."

— **MEG, age 57**

"I've always loved music and dancing. I can be in a foul mood, but when I get in my car, turn on the radio or pop in a CD and just go for a drive, music immediately picks me up. I'm also a crier, and that seems to help release frustration. It also helps me to talk about it, especially with the person who angered me—after I cool down."

— **Paulette, age 59**

"I use meditation, yoga, active exercise, Mindfulness-Based Stress Reduction (MBSR) tools, or even knitting as I sit and center on what I'm doing."

— **Babs, age 66**

"I've really made a concerted effort to release anger. I was raised in a Catholic family with five children, and we had one major rule: everyone must get along! Feeling anger wasn't something that was ever encouraged, and I grew up feeling that it was beneath me. Apparently, however, pouting and implosions were okay, as that's what I did more often. But when I learned how to heal my anxieties and fears, I decided to handle this type of stress better. I now use 'I messages' to deal with upsets. I also use 'When you did/said this, I felt this,'

type of communication. This places me less in a victim mentality and more in an empowered state of mind. The point is to express yourself in an effective way, not necessarily to control the person who angered or upset you. Venting is its own reward when done to release the hurt."

— **Kathryn, age 59**

Anger and negativity are like dust on the furniture or dirt on your clothes. They have to be removed regularly. And although the process isn't always enjoyable, how wonderful it is to don fresh, clean clothes—or walk into a newly cleaned room. Now it's your turn to start dusting!

My Personal Action Plan for Pleasure:
Releasing Anger and Negativity

The following are warning signs I can learn to watch out for that flag anger and negativity coming on (such as recurrent negative thoughts or unconscious habits, including overeating, racing heartbeat, or even bouts of clumsiness):

1. _____

2. _____

3. _____

Situations that often bring on negativity that I can avoid:

1. _____

2. _____

3. _____

My exit plan for dealing with anger and negativity:

_____

_____

_____

_____

_____

I commit to regularly noticing and releasing my anger and negativity.

_____

(Signature)

_____

(Date)

6

Commit to Regularly Exploring Your Body's Pleasure Potential

*J*ust as it's important to practice self-pleasuring on a regular basis, if you have a partner, you must also commit to frequently exploring your sensuality together if you want the steamiest sex life possible.

Don't make it all about intercourse—and don't even make your goal orgasm. Just commit to feeling as much pleasure as possible and becoming comfortable giving instructions and talking about what you like in bed. (Offering positive feedback every time your partner does something right is an excellent start.) See how the following women keep their romance alive, passion primed, and lovemaking luscious.

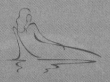

"In my marriage of 15 years, I've always worried if I was pleasing my husband. But something has totally changed inside me in the last year, and it's been scary and exciting at the same time! Our sex life was always good, but now it's fantastic. Sex isn't just sex anymore; it has so much more meaning. I concentrate on my own pleasure. I'm doing it for me now because I enjoy it—not because I think I'm supposed to. I've found that having a voice in what gives me pleasure has made my marriage so much stronger. I feel more confident as a woman in all areas of my life."

— **Nicole, age 37**

"By taking responsibility for my own sexual pleasure, I found that I'm more loving and gentle even with myself. I also tell my partner that I love him often. He is a gentle man, and he gives me a foot and leg massage every night. I love that."

— **Janice, age 56**

"After 35 years of marriage, it's easier to talk about sex, so our sex life is much better now. One of the best ways I've found to keep romance going is to be thoughtful. I make my husband's favorite dinner, light some candles, and we watch a good romantic movie. It works."

— **Irene, age 61**

"We make dates with each other, usually earlier in the day or the day before. This helps the anticipation build, and by the time we're alone, we're really ready for each other! I enjoy sex *so* much more in midlife. The reason is because I've learned to stop feeling guilty or bad for wanting pleasure. Although this is a work in progress, I'm starting to speak up and say what I like and don't like. Learning to trust my partner and ask for what I want has been liberating. I can't say that I'm totally comfortable yet, but things are *much* better than they were, say, five years ago."

— **Lynn, age 53**

"I write a love note on the napkin that I put in my husband's lunch bag. I bless him every night and morning. We give full-body hugs without clothes on . . . in the kitchen."
— **Kathy, age 57**

"I definitely enjoy sex now more than ever. I know myself and my body so much better, and I'm not afraid to tell my partner what pleases me. Speak up, ladies! You'll be surprised that your partner really does want to know what to do. I definitely take more responsibility for my own pleasure. I no longer am afraid of what people will think or if I'm a 'bad girl' for wanting a certain thing. My mate is more than happy to oblige me."
— **DD, age 43**

"We exchange a text message, e-mail, or phone call that just says, 'Love you.' And we still plan our date nights even though we're empty nesters. We also give

a pinch here and there or a quick hug!"
— **Robin, age 51**

"I do special things for him that he likes, and we also just sit together in the evenings and talk about our day. Then I ask him to rub my back. It always leads to more! I buy such beautiful undies and keep my body smelling so good! Steamy sex is being spontaneous—anywhere, anytime! I know what I want now and say it. And I don't settle, ever. I say *stop* if it doesn't feel great and share what would feel better. He loves that I share what I want, so he doesn't have to play a guessing game."
— **Pamila, age 49**

"We have great conversations about what we find most pleasing. After 40 years, we can talk about anything. Our relationship is very close, and we have lots of fun together. We're best friends, and we laugh a lot."
— **Carol, age 62**

"As I feel more confident, I enjoy sex more. I know what I like—what turns me on and what doesn't. It isn't all about my guy anymore. It's a lot more about what I like. I think men like foreplay as much as women do. Men like a woman who initiates something, even if it's just asking for a date. Showers and baths for two have always been a hit, as well as both giving and getting massages. Having similar likes but also having other interests keeps romance alive. Being sensitive to the relationship is very important, as is keeping constant vigilance. Don't fall asleep, so to speak, where your mate is concerned."

— **NKM, age 52**

"My husband never ceases to surprise and delight me because he's so good at finding pleasure points on my body that I never even knew were there. We're very ideas oriented. Sometimes we spontaneously massage each other—which we're both good at—and end up having wonderful sex. But at other times, we play around with ideas and talk about them. If we have a bottle of champagne that's been in the fridge for weeks, we might decide to pick up some large, fresh, yummy shrimp with special sauce at a favorite food place of ours. We'll fill a lovely wine chiller with ice and put the champagne bottle in it. Then we'll bring that and the shrimp platter into the bedroom, set it on a cocktail table, tell each other sexy stories, sip champagne, and have sex—not necessarily in that order. We've used that one twice, and we're looking forward to number three! It's a 'delicious' experience on many levels."

— **Linda, age 56**

"Sex is so much more enjoyable when we share what we prefer. Keeping an open mind about trying something new or playing out each other's fantasies are wonderful expressions of caring about our partners and ourselves."

— **Elizabeth, age 55**

"My current companion is the hottest, sexiest, most devilish thing; and I have a hard time keeping my hands to myself. He does, too. He's the most romantic person I know. I'm so responsive to his touch, and it's a big turn-on for me to observe his reactions. I enjoy being with him so much that even if I don't reach orgasm, it doesn't matter. Because I was brought up with 12 children and a strict religious background, it was hard to break the chains that bind, but break them I did! I've overcome my guilt and am now trying to tell my companion what I like and how. He's very attentive and wants to please me. Sometimes it's easy to verbalize, and sometimes it's not. It's probably the most difficult thing to do, but if I want intimacy, I have to do this. You can't fake it."

— **Randy, age 77**

"I love my husband and spend quality time talking to him, looking him in the eyes, and listening to him. He notices when I change my nail-polish color, and I notice when he trims his beard. After 19 years, we'd stopped seeing each other. But we've found our sight again."

— **Katherine, age 47**

"I lucked out by finding a man who took it upon himself at an early age to actually study what pleases women. (He took a sexuality class in college, I think.) I can't imagine being intimate with anyone else. We let each other know when we want to have sex in or out of the bedroom, and we're very open as to what we want to do in terms of positions and so on. We've tried using sex toys, but we actually don't like them—especially vibrators, which I find too harsh, too buzzy, and too distracting."

— **Claudia, age 57**

"I enjoy sex in a different way now because it's attached to a loving partner. We are accepting, open, and passionate with each other; and when we go away without the kids—*yow!* I'm much more open now and can tell my husband anything I want, and he tells me what he wants, too. I can also tell him what works for me and what doesn't. We have sex quite regularly, and it's always good. (Even when we're tired and just have a quickie, it's still a great release!) Sometimes he likes it when I pleasure myself while he's inside me, which can be really exciting."

— **Barbara, age 54**

"It's important to take special time for sex; it keeps us close and connected. We sometimes go off to Miami Beach for a night or have a nice evening walk on the beach. Our mellow caring and love works for us! We also leave each other romantic cards in the morning by the coffeepot. 'Hello' phone calls are a daily routine."

— **Valerie, age 56**

"He never knows what to expect from me. You have to keep the mystique in a marriage, no matter how long you've been together. You also need to let your man know that he's the greatest thing since chocolate."

— **Paulette, age 59**

"When I want sex, I'm comfortable initiating it. I know my body much better now, and I know what my partner needs to do to please me. I give him feedback without seeming demanding. I think he tries harder to please me when I do speak up, so it's a win-win."
— **Barb, age 47**

"My husband constantly tells me that I'm as gorgeous as the day we met—18 years ago!"
— **Michele, age 50**

"I love the fact that there are so many options for pleasure, besides just having intercourse. Watching a good porno film is always fun—a little corny sometimes, but it sure helps put you in the mood. Toys are also enjoyable when I'm having a wild thought or two. My husband is very accommodating to my ups and downs in moods. A relaxing back massage will usually result in some intimacy. The more I have sex, the more I want it. It's known that the chemicals produced during an orgasm actually help keep you attracted to your mate.

When all is in sync with my husband, I feel an overall satisfaction with the world as a whole. I seem to be a better parent, friend, and lover. I love sex!"
— Lisa, age 45

"Since I've reawakened to myself as a sexual being, I'm increasingly aware of my role as a channel through which sacred energy enters the universe. My husband now worships me in our lovemaking in a way that I think is only possible between two people who've gone the distance together and know and trust each other deeply. Most of our sexual encounters begin with his giving me oral sex, including using his fingers inside of me, for a very long time! At first this desire to service me so generously on a regular basis made me very uncomfortable. Relaxing enough to really receive this type of raw, undiluted pleasure was a challenge! But once I connected what he was asking of me to this image of myself as a conduit of sacred energy, I began to relax. He says it gives him enormous pleasure to see me having one orgasm after another. It's as if he's drinking from a source that's only available to him through me.

The heights of pleasure that I experience as his mastery of what pleases me surpasses my own is intense! By the time he releases me and we have intercourse, I'm as open to him as I possibly could be and take him in more deeply than I would be able to otherwise. The power of having him in me in this way spins us both to places and to a connection that the word *spiritual* only begins to describe."

— **Sarah, age 44**

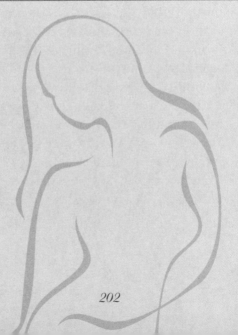

Remember, your body was designed to experience unlimited pleasure—and when you allow yourself to experience this, you're helping uplift the entire world. How exciting!

My Personal Action Plan for Pleasure:
Regularly Exploring My Pleasure Potential

What I most appreciate about my partner:

1. _____

2. _____

3. _____

Ways that I can emotionally reconnect with my partner and express how much I appreciate him or her:

1. _____

2. _____

3. _____

What I'd like to experiment with or try with my partner to dial up our sensual and sexual pleasure (including giving feedback in bed):

1. _____

2. _____

3. _____

I now commit to regularly exploring my pleasure potential with my partner as I've outlined here.

_____

(Signature)

_____

(Date)

7

Live Your Life in a Way That Excites, Motivates, and "Turns On" Others to Be at Their Best—and Healthiest

hy not inspire the people around you to reach for joy themselves? Better yet, why not become a *source* of pleasure for others? I recommend giving frequent praise and noting when an individual does something right. Become adept at what I call the "drive-by compliment" with all sorts of people, including those you don't know! As the following women attest, the more pleasure you spread to others, the more pleasure you'll feel yourself—and the more joyous and healthy the world around you will become. Try it!

"Sometimes, when a young mother is behind me in line at the grocery store, I tell the checker to put her items on my bill."
— **Janice, age 56**

"I hope that my living example will help other women around me see that age is just a number and attitude is everything. When I'm giving a massage to a client, I imagine that I'm an open channel for universal love and light. I visualize this love and light streaming through my hands and filling the individuals I'm working on. I ask the universe to give these people only what they need, and I try not to project onto them what I think they may need. I see each person as a beautiful, shiny soul, full of purity and light. I also make sure to thank people who extend kindnesses to me, such as opening a door, waiting on me in a restaurant, or letting me over in traffic; and I always try to do these things for others. I'll even look at strangers in a store and smile and make eye contact."
— **Lynn, age 53**

"I've given myself permission to watch more movies, read more, look out the window at nature and the birds at my feeders, or to just sit and be, allowing myself to do as I please without *any* guilty feelings at all. I've been sharing my new philosophy with other women I come in contact with, whether at the post office, grocery store, or at my twice-a-month fellowship lunches. Most of the women I talk to have *no* idea how to give themselves permission to receive more pleasure or even why they should do so. But I'm making progress planting those seeds of thought in their spirits. It's been very rewarding for me to see others begin to incorporate my suggestions. I like to believe that I'm helping set other women free . . . emotionally and otherwise."

— **Martha**, age 57

"I'm trying to make a real effort each day to be a source of happiness, joy, and peace for people in every interaction I have. I challenge myself to try to make others smile and be glad that they talked to me. I look for those I like or want to be like—people with a joyful,

loving, or happy expression—and I try to learn more about them."
— **Kimberli, age 52**

"I always see something good in others, and I compliment them on it. We hear enough negative words in our daily lives. I think it's refreshing to look for the positive, and it surprises people these days to receive a kind word out of the blue, unsolicited. They beam, and I think it lifts them, carrying them through the rest of their day. At least I hope so. It does for me! I work for a major airline, and I frequently hear complaints. Thank-yous are, well, not heard very often; and when they do surface, it's just in passing. But when someone looks me in the eye and says, 'Thank you,' I'm so impressed. It stays in my memory because it's sincere. Simple but genuine social graces go a long way."
— **NKM, age 52**

"I am a beautiful, smiling, truly happy woman in a wheelchair, with no complaints. People who see me at my fitness center, at the supermarket, or in a museum often stop me and say, 'You're such an inspiration to me!' But I'm just living my life, trying to get from point A to B. Just being who I am, as I am, has forced many people to make a quick attitude adjustment when they see me. It always astounds and pleases me when it happens, because even after 28 years of this, I don't expect it. It makes others realize that anything is possible. Just stop complaining, and *do it*."

— **Linda, age 56**

"It's been my experience that when you feel joy, everyone wants a piece of it. It's about being nonjudgmental and open to allowing others to be themselves and try new things that feel good. It's also about allowing people to know that they have a safe place to talk about anything and that it will be okay."

— **Elizabeth, age 55**

"After having a heart-valve replacement at 76, I found that I had more energy and determination than ever. I wanted to fulfill my dream of finishing a degree that I started 26 years ago, so I enrolled at the local community college. In spite of needing cataracts removed, I got an A in my first drawing course. I also work part-time, and to my amazement, I find that many co-workers and managers see me as their role model. I work at Disney, where the combination of my energy, enthusiasm, and imagination are the inspiration to many menopausal women as well as younger ones. My children, grandchildren, and great-grandchildren don't know what to think, but my brothers and sisters, my co-workers, and everyone else I know are so proud and in awe. Working to pay my tuition only adds to their accolades."

— **Randy, age 77**

"I'm known as the 'social director' among my girlfriends. When I decided to make a quilt for my daughter and her husband, I got some of my girlfriends involved in their own projects. We go away for the weekend two to four times a year to work on our crafts. Almost five years later, I'm still working on that quilt. I also give my friends little gifts for no reason other than because I know it's something they like. This can be just a little notepad or a fan (for those midlife power surges). I make cards for all occasions, and my friends really appreciate them. I also think they know that I'm always there for them. They can ask for my help and support anytime, and I offer it often before they have a chance to ask."

— **Claudia**, age 57

"I smile at people. I try to be positive, and it seems to help others be positive, too. I give praise to those who deserve it. I thank everyone who helps me, no matter how small the way. I address people by name if I know it (name badges help a lot), and I let them know how much I appreciate them."

— **Diane**, age 51

"I like to smile at strangers, and I believe in the chain reaction of smiles and random kindness."
— **Valerie, age 56**

"I write notes to tell people how much I appreciate them."
— **Kathy, age 57**

"I smile all the time. It's infectious. People always comment on my high energy and upbeat personality. I laugh the loudest at myself. I'm a riot!"
— **Dana, age 58**

"My guiding principle is to connect with people as often as possible. I practice this by really looking at them and listening to them and by focusing all of my attention on their words, their meaning, and their experiences. In this way, I hope that I help others feel

valued and validated so that they will, in turn, have the energy to do this for others in their lives."
— **Colleen, age 45**

"I start every day thinking that I'm going to say something to make someone feel better about him- or herself. It brings me joy as well!"
— **Irene, age 61**

"I do good things when no one is looking."
— **Pat, age 63**

"I believe that when we live our life 'out loud'— embracing who we are, where we are—we can't help but inspire others. Being unapologetically exuberant, with an ear-to-ear smile on my face, and fully embracing my beauty spreads joy. For years I thought I was fat, ugly, and stupid, but those were old, invalid tapes that I've destroyed. In their place, I realized that I'm a knockout, a gifted writer, and a skilled artist. I've even found a way to make a living helping other women see their own beauty in a gentle, accepting, nurturing environment of my own creation. In sharing my story of triumph over trauma, I inspire others to believe that they can be triumphant, too. My clients give me feedback on a daily basis about how I've touched their lives. I'm so very, very blessed! And I know that I wouldn't be where I am today, nor would I be in the position to help as many women as I do, had I *not* had the challenges to overcome that I did. It didn't kill me—although sometimes it felt as if it would—and I'm stronger, kinder, and more beautiful than ever because of it. It was an inside job."

— BD, age 48

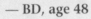

This section reminds me of the theme song from the 1970s television hit *The Mary Tyler Moore Show*—are *you* ready to turn the world on with your smile? Well, now it's your turn!

My Personal Action Plan for Pleasure:
Uplifting and Turning On Others

I joyously commit to "turning on" the world around me (including both people I know and complete strangers who cross my path) in the following ways:

1. _____

2. _____

3. _____

4. _____

5. _____

Volunteer opportunities I'd like to pursue:

1. _____

2. _____

3. _____

I now commit to taking at least one action a day that uplifts someone else.

_____

(Signature)

_____

(Date)

Afterword

*C*ongratulations! You've created your own personal blueprint for transforming your life and your health through the discipline of pleasure. Yes, it's a discipline. Remember this: nothing is easier than slipping into negativity. Our culture thrives on it. Just watch the news.

But you have the power of choice. And now you have all the tools and inspiration you'll ever need to turn yourself on with the health-enhancing benefits of nitric-oxide-producing pleasure—any time, any place.

Here's what I recommend: keep this book on your bedside table. Begin your day by reading through just one or two pages so that you can start off feeling and expecting more pleasure. Keep looking for more and more ways to experience pleasure and spread it around. This ignites the positive upward spiral of health in your body.

Better yet, gather a group of friends and work on upping your pleasure potential together. Meet weekly or monthly—whatever time allows. Or form a group on the Internet, where you can post your continuing adventures in flourishing through pleasure. We all love hearing how someone prevailed over sadness, anger, or despair—and then went on to create something truly joyful! There's nothing like a group of women really going for it to keep you inspired. And there's nothing more fun than listening to the triumphs of others who are daring to live with more pleasure.

Yes, this takes courage. It takes guts. But you have nothing to lose by following this path—except illness and pain. Over time the journey gets easier, especially because you'll be surrounding yourself with those who are doing the same thing. Remember the old saying: dimming your light in order to make others more comfortable makes the whole world darker. *You were meant to shine!* You were meant to be a source of delight for yourself and others. So shine on, dear one. Shine on!

— Christiane Northrup, M.D.

Acknowledgments

A huge thank-you to all the women who contributed their heartwarming, hot, and health-enhancing stories in this volume—as a gift of inspiration for their sisters.

And also to Katy Koontz who, after working on the original *Secret Pleasures of Menopause,* said to me, "It would be great to have some more specific instructions for women on how to actually increase pleasure in their lives. The nitty-gritty details." And I said, "Good idea." Thank you, Katy, for the inspiration—and also for the artful way you helped collect and edit these juicy pleasure instructions.

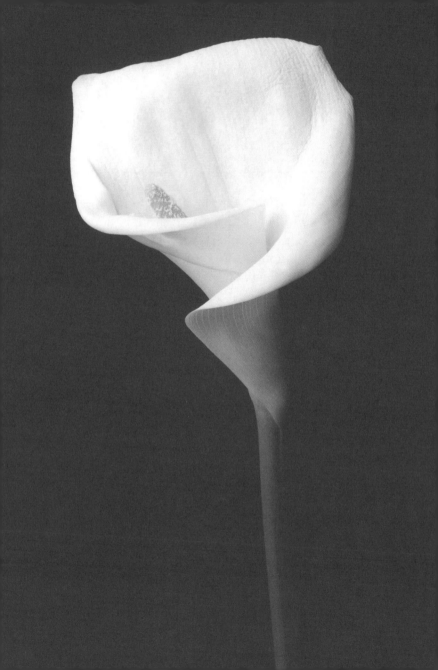

About the Author

*C*hristiane Northrup, M.D., is a visionary pioneer and beloved authority in the field of women's health and wellness. A board-certified ob-gyn who graduated from Dartmouth Medical School and did her residency at Tufts–New England Medical Center, Dr. Northrup was also an assistant clinical professor of obstetrics-gynecology at Maine Medical Center for more than 20 years. Recognizing the unity of body, mind, and spirit, she helps empower women to tune in to their innate inner wisdom in order to truly flourish on all levels.

Dr. Northrup is the author of two *New York Times* best-selling books, *Women's Bodies, Women's Wisdom* and *The Wisdom of Menopause.* Her third book, *Mother-Daughter Wisdom,* was a 2005 Quill Award nominee and was voted **Amazon.com**'s number one book of the year in both Parenting and Mind/Body Health. In 2008, she published her fourth major book, *The Secret Pleasures of Menopause.*

Dr. Northrup has also hosted six highly successful PBS specials. Her latest, *Menopause and Beyond: New Wisdom for Women,* began airing nationwide in March 2007. Her work has been featured on *The Oprah Winfrey Show,* the *Today* show, *NBC Nightly News with Tom Brokaw, The View, Rachael Ray,* and *Good Morning America.*

For more information about Dr. Northrup and her work, please visit her Website at: **www.drnorthrup.com**.

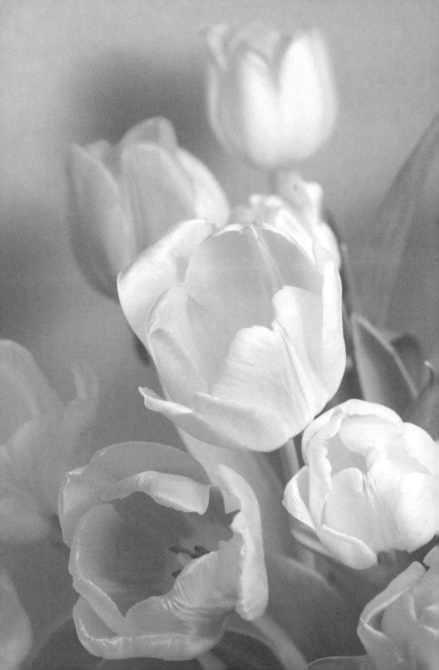

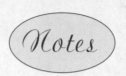

Notes

_____

_____

_____

_____

_____

_____

_____

_____

_____

_____

_____

_____

_____

_____

_____

_____

_____

Notes

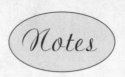

Notes

_____

_____

_____

_____

_____

_____

_____

_____

_____

_____

_____

_____

_____

_____

_____

_____

_____

_____

Notes

Hay House Titles of Related Interest

YOU CAN HEAL YOUR LIFE, the movie,
starring Louise L. Hay & Friends
(available as a 1-DVD program and an expanded 2-DVD set)
Watch the trailer at: **www.LouiseHayMovie.com**

AMBITION TO MEANING: Finding Your Life's Purpose, the movie,
starring Dr. Wayne W. Dyer
(available as a 1-DVD program and an expanded 2-DVD set)
Watch the trailer at: **www.DyerMovie.com**

THE AGE OF MIRACLES: Embracing the New Midlife,
by Marianne Williamson

***THE ART OF EXTREME SELF-CARE: Transform Your Life
One Month at a Time,*** by Cheryl Richardson

***THE BODY KNOWS . . . HOW TO STAY YOUNG: Healthy-Aging
Secrets from a Medical Intuitive,*** by Caroline Sutherland

***EMPOWERING WOMEN: Every Woman's Guide
to Successful Living,*** by Louise L. Hay

REPOTTING: 10 Steps for Redesigning Your Life,
by Diana Holman and Ginger Pape

***SIMPLY . . . WOMAN! The 12-Week Body-Mind-Soul Total
Transformation Program,*** by Crystal Andrus

***SQUEEZE THE DAY: 365 Ways to Bring Joy
and Juice into Your Life,*** by Loretta LaRoche

All of the above are available at your local bookstore,
or may be ordered by contacting Hay House (see next page).

We hope you enjoyed this Hay House book. If you'd like to receive a free catalog featuring additional Hay House books and products, or if you'd like information about the Hay Foundation, please contact:

Hay House, Inc.
P.O. Box 5100
Carlsbad, CA 92018-5100

(760) 431-7695 or **(800) 654-5126**
(760) 431-6948 (fax) or **(800) 650-5115 (fax)**
www.hayhouse.com® • **www.hayfoundation.org**

Published and distributed in Australia by: Hay House Australia Pty. Ltd., 18/36 Ralph St., Alexandria NSW 2015 • *Phone:* 612-9669-4299 *Fax:* 612-9669-4144 • www.hayhouse.com.au

Published and distributed in the United Kingdom by: Hay House UK, Ltd., 292B Kensal Rd., London W10 5BE • *Phone:* 44-20-8962-1230 *Fax:* 44-20-8962-1239 • www.hayhouse.co.uk

Published and distributed in the Republic of South Africa by: Hay House SA (Pty), Ltd., P.O. Box 990, Witkoppen 2068 • *Phone/Fax:* 27-11-467-8904 • orders@psdprom.co.za • www.hayhouse.co.za

Published in India by: Hay House Publishers India, Muskaan Complex, Plot No. 3, B-2, Vasant Kunj, New Delhi 110 070 • *Phone:* 91-11-4176-1620 • *Fax:* 91-11-4176-1630 • www.hayhouse.co.in

Distributed in Canada by: Raincoast, 9050 Shaughnessy St., Vancouver, B.C. V6P 6E5 • *Phone:* (604) 323-7100 • *Fax:* (604) 323-2600 www.raincoast.com

Tune in to **HayHouseRadio.com®** for the best in inspirational talk radio featuring top Hay House authors! And, sign up via the Hay House USA Website to receive the Hay House online newsletter and stay informed about what's going on with your favorite authors. You'll receive bimonthly announcements about Discounts and Offers, Special Events, Product Highlights, Free Excerpts, Giveaways, and more!
www.hayhouse.com®